Acupuncture for Chronic Pelvic Pain in Women

of related interest

Cultivating a Sustainable Core
A Framework Integrating Body, Mind, and Breath
into Musculoskeletal Rehabilitation
Liz Gillem Duncanson
Foreword by Shelly Prosko
ISBN 978 1 78775 420 1
eISBN 978 1 78775 421 8

Pelvic Rehabilitation
The Manual Therapy and Exercise Guide Across the Lifespan
Maureen Mason
Foreword by Ginger Garner
ISBN 978 1 91342 609 5
eISBN 978 1 91342 610 1

Pelvic Yoga Therapy for the Whole Woman
A Professional Guide
Cheri Dostal Ryba
Foreword by Shelly Prosko and Eve Andry
ISBN 978 1 78775 664 9
eISBN 978 1 78775 665 6

Acupuncture for Chronic Pelvic Pain in Women

Ooi Thye Chong

Foreword by Lorie Eve Dechar

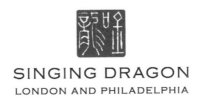

SINGING DRAGON
LONDON AND PHILADELPHIA

First published in Great Britain in 2024 by Singing Dragon,
an imprint of Jessica Kingsley Publishers
Part of John Murray Press

1

Copyright © Ooi Thye Chong 2024
Foreword copyright © Lorie Eve Dechar 2024

The right of Ooi Thye Chong to be identified as the Author of the Work has been
asserted by her in accordance with the Copyright, Designs and Patents Act 1988.

Front cover illustration source: Masha Pimas.

All rights reserved. No part of this publication may be reproduced, stored in a retrieval system,
or transmitted, in any form or by any means without the prior written permission of the
publisher, nor be otherwise circulated in any form of binding or cover other than that in which
it is published and without a similar condition being imposed on the subsequent purchaser.

A CIP catalogue record for this title is available from the
British Library and the Library of Congress

ISBN 978 1 78775 847 6
eISBN 978 1 78775 848 3

Printed and bound in the United States by Integrated Books International

Jessica Kingsley Publishers' policy is to use papers that are natural, renewable and recyclable
products and made from wood grown in sustainable forests. The logging and manufacturing
processes are expected to conform to the environmental regulations of the country of origin.

Singing Dragon
Carmelite House
50 Victoria Embankment
London EC4Y 0DZ

www.singingdragon.com

John Murray Press
Part of Hodder & Stoughton Limited
An Hachette UK Company

To Jeff who loves, nurtures and nourishes.

Contents

Acknowledgements 9

Foreword by Lorie Eve Dechar 11

Preface 13

1. Introduction 15

2. Chronic Pelvic Pain in Women 25

3. The Local Balance Method 45

4. The Global Balance Method 69

5. Trigger Points 93

6. Five Elements Theory-Based Acupuncture Treatment 117

7. An Alchemical Healing Approach to Transforming
   Psycho-Emotional Distress 143

8. Nurturing and Nourishing Ourselves: Chinese Medicine
   Approach to Food 163

9. Creating a Toolbox to Nurture and Nourish Ourselves . . . 185

References 203

Endnotes 211

Index 213

Acknowledgements

Many years ago, I expressed to my then boyfriend (who would become my husband), Professor Jeffrey Pollard, a long-held desire to obtain a university education, an ambition that could not be fulfilled because I believed that I was not 'clever' or good enough. His encouraging and positive response played a fundamental role in my continued quest for knowledge and to be the best that I can be. Thank you for believing in me.

My profound gratitude to Benjamin Fox and Lorie Eve Dechar for their infinite wisdom, valuable comments and encouragement, and their willingness to lend me their support. Thank you also to Rea Mattocks and Dr Nina Shoulberg, who painstakingly read each chapter, gave me their honest opinions, and corrected my grammar.

I am also indebted to Dr Andrew Horne, Dr Delphine Armand, Dr Diane Rooney and Dr Bianca Beldini, who generously gave their time and their expert opinions. Also, a heart-felt thank you to Dr Wai Nyin and Dr Wolfgang Wald, who provided insightful contributions to the book.

Last, but not least, a hat tip to the editorial director Claire Wilson and her team in bringing the book to fruition.

Foreword

There is a web of wisdom being woven by women engaged in the holistic healing of other women that is rapidly growing in rigour, depth, substance and clinical efficacy. This web brings together practitioners and scholars in the fields of traditional Chinese medicine, somatic and depth psychology, gynaecology and trauma studies as well as ecology, consciousness exploration and cultural transformation. The web is dedicated to the alleviation of the suffering of women and a deepening of our understanding of feminine psychology; however, at its core the web is also part of a redemption of the sacredness of the feminine principle, a redemption that touches every human being regardless of gender, and that has an impact on the very future of our planet.

With the publication of this impeccably researched, painstakingly organized, and clinically relevant guidebook, Dr Ooi Thye Chong joins the ranks of these wisdom weavers as she offers us a new way of approaching entrenched pain and suffering at the most vulnerable and intimate level of a woman's body. This book brings together Dr Chong's many decades of experience in both Western and Chinese medicine. It is a passionate, intelligent and welcome antidote to the predominant Western medical view that minimizes women's pelvic pain to a purely physical problem. With its solid grounding in Western and Taoist philosophy, as well as its diagnostic precision, clearly described treatment strategies, detailed case studies and personal writing style, the book pioneers a new paradigm for the treatment of chronic pelvic pain while also being of immediate clinical value to acupuncturists who are working with women with chronic pelvic pain as well as a wide range of practitioners of other modalities.

Dr Chong's method offers a multifaceted approach that has proven to have lasting effectiveness on physical and psychological levels while avoiding the side effects of medications and the various challenges of surgery. It combines Chinese medicine with potent yet doable non-needling skills, including visualization, Meditation, affirmations and active imagination, which touch the subtle, non-physical aspects of pelvic pain. But, most importantly, the book brings a new respect to the complexity of chronic pelvic pain in women, and highlights the care and compassion as well as the wide variety of clinical tools required for its successful treatment.

I am honoured to have been in conversation with Dr Chong as she worked over many years to develop, refine and articulate her method. It is no surprise to me that the curious, creative, fiercely dedicated healer I met in 2003 as my student at the Tri-State College of Acupuncture in New York has developed this elegant, synergistic approach, and I am proud to have been able to offer my support along the way.

My own life has been graced and illuminated by knowing Dr Chong, first as a student and mentee, and now as an inspired colleague and treasured friend. I have no doubt that this book will be an inspiration and a treasure to those who seek to move beyond the masking of symptoms, to heal not only the branches but also the root cause of a widespread and debilitating chronic disease. In honouring the mystery and depth as well as the transformational potential of this suffering that afflicts hundreds of thousands of women across the globe, Dr Chong earns her place as a true Alchemical Healer, an astute analyst of empirical evidence and medical theory, as well as an artisan of the life force and a physician of the soul.

Lorie Eve Dechar

Preface

This book was conceived after I witnessed the distress some of my patients with chronic pelvic pain experienced, and how they responded positively to the different acupuncture treatments they received from me. I am therefore excited to share my professional experience with traditionally trained acupuncturists working with women who suffer from chronic pelvic pain and other healthcare professionals who are interested. The book will also be useful for those who want to use a non-drug approach to managing pain.

The book has nine chapters. The physical approach to pain management is explored in Chapters 3, 4 and 5, and the psycho-emotional approach in Chapters 6 and 7. Chapters 8 and 9 focus on how we can take care of ourselves using food and practices such as Yoga, Qi Gong and Breathwork.

Chapter 1 gives an overview of the physical and psycho-emotional approaches to managing chronic pelvic pain in women. Chronic pelvic pain is a complex and challenging condition that biomedicine has not been able to treat satisfactorily. Thus, I have included Dr Richard Teh-Fu Tan's Balance Method (BM) acupuncture and trigger point deactivation, Five Elements acupuncture and Alchemical Healing, as well as tools for self-care.

Chapter 2 describes the clinical background, possible causes and challenges of chronic pelvic pain in women. I begin with an overview of chronic pelvic pain – its financial, social and emotional impact on the lives of women as well as its standard medical and surgical management. This chapter also draws attention to the lack of satisfactory biomedical standard management of chronic pelvic pain.

Chapter 3 focuses on Local Balance Method acupuncture. I have included a step-by-step instruction for using the method, which involves the Five Systems and Mirror and Image Methods for point selection as well as case studies.

Chapter 4 presents the Global Balance Method. It differentiates Static Balance from Dynamic Balance as well as the Local Balance Method from the Global Balance Method. This chapter also highlights the different indications for using the Global Balance Method.

Chapter 5 explains what trigger points are, and gives an overview of the most common trigger points that may be responsible for or contribute to chronic pelvic pain in women. It guides the reader to deactivating trigger points using classical Chinese acupuncture.

Chapter 6 gives an overview of the Five Elements theory and its importance in understanding the psycho-emotional aspects of both our patients and ourselves. It outlines common Five Elements treatment protocols for emotional blocks.

Chapter 7 presents Alchemical Healing where needling and non-needling methods are used to heal and transform psycho-emotional distress and chaos.

Chapter 8 focuses on how we can nourish and nurture ourselves and offer women with chronic pelvic pain advice using food as medicine.

Chapter 9 emphasizes the importance of self-care through different practices that focus on Breathwork, such as Yoga, Tai Chi, Qi Gong and Meditation.

—— CHAPTER 1 ——

INTRODUCTION

This book is written for professional acupuncturists and healthcare professionals working with women who suffer from chronic pelvic pain. You will learn several different styles of acupuncture and non-needling tools to help relieve your patients' pain so they feel a whole lot better. When working with women who are in pain, there are many useful practical tips that can be imparted to help them be actively involved in their own care, so they can regain some power and agency over their own life: 'For people who live with chronic pain, this seeps into all facets of their life like a slow poison. It disables one function after another, switches off mental and emotional connections and corrupts all the rules of life' (Chan 2019).

Chronic pelvic pain in women is more common than we think. Its worldwide prevalence is estimated to range from between 5.7 and 26.6 per cent (Ahangari 2014). In the UK primary care setting, 38 out of 1000 women were found to have chronic pelvic pain (Zondervan *et al.* 1999). Chronic pelvic pain is often associated with gynaecological conditions (endometriosis), gastrointestinal conditions (e.g., irritable bowel syndrome, IBS) and urinary conditions (painful bladder syndrome, PBS) as well as trigger points that are tight and sensitive areas in the skeletal muscle. Characteristically, trigger points produce local and referred pain as well as a twitch response when palpated (Simons, Travell and Simons 1999). A significant number of these women have severe painful menstruation and/or pain during sexual intercourse, urination or defecation. These constellations of problems negatively impact on their quality of life. Additionally, chronic pelvic pain is intimately associated with psycho-emotional factors (depression, sleep disturbance, anxiety), making it an extremely complex and challenging condition to treat and manage. This highly complex picture is consistently mirrored in the women I treat. It is fair to say that standard biomedicine approaches to managing chronic pelvic pain are not satisfactory as they often have unacceptable and unwanted side effects, even if some strategies are helpful for the pain.

The present book is born out of this urgent need for an effective approach that has little or no unwanted and unacceptable side effects. Because of the complexity and challenging nature of chronic pelvic pain, I have integrated several different important and effective non-drug approaches to dealing with the physical and psycho-emotional aspects of pain. The physical approaches are based on Dr Tan's Balance Method (BM) acupuncture and the classical acupuncture method to deactivate trigger points. Additionally, I am excited to present some psycho-emotional approaches, which include Five Elements acupuncture and Lorie Eve Dechar's Alchemical Healing.

The physical and psycho-emotional approaches of taking care of patients seems comprehensive, albeit rather incomplete, if the patient is not actively encouraged to be involved in their own health. I firmly believe that 'doing things for the patient' is enhanced when they are actively involved in their own care. This book will therefore help practitioners to introduce to women suffering from chronic pelvic pain the many ways they can take care of themselves and regain some control over their own bodies. The same can be applied to ourselves as health-care practitioners, for we must also remember to tend to our own needs so that we are in a sound physical and psycho-emotional state to be able to care for others. Thus, I have included two very important and essential chapters on nurturing and nourishing ourselves (see Chapters 8 and 9).

INTRODUCTION

MY FIRST ENCOUNTERS WITH BALANCE METHOD ACUPUNCTURE

I discovered Balance Method (BM) acupuncture through a chance remark made by a fellow student about the late Dr Tan's style, which produced instant pain relief. Dr Tan used to call BM acupuncture 'Acupuncture 1, 2, 3'. In trying to relieve pain in patients who had not responded to traditional Chinese acupuncture, I studied and then applied Dr Tan's methods to these patients. What follows are their stories.

A patient with a sore right thumb, who had shown no reduction in pain with traditional acupuncture, was treated following Dr Tan's BM acupuncture. One needle was inserted into an Ashi point (tight and tender point) of her left big toe. As soon as the needle was inserted, she reported a reduction in pain. I repeated the steps outlined by Dr Tan until her pain was reduced by a good 90 per cent. Like most people who had first encountered or heard of the immediate pain relief of BM acupuncture, I must admit that I was incredulous. I was convinced that it was all a placebo affect, that the pain relief was due to other causes rather than the acupuncture treatment. But there she was, smiling at me and showing me that her thumb had more mobility and hardly any pain, which was a vast improvement on the last treatment. She needed several more treatments to fully recover.

Shortly after this very exciting experience, I treated another patient with BM acupuncture. She was a patient at a cancer centre in New York City, where I worked for many years. This patient had had a bilateral mastectomy for breast cancer with a TRAM (transverse rectus abdominis muscle) flap breast reconstruction (a piece of skin, fat and all or part of the underlying rectus abdominis muscle (our 'six pack') was used to reconstruct the breast). She was about 10 days post-operation when she had her first appointment with me. At that point, she was in considerable pain as the prescribed pain medications had not been helpful. When she entered my treatment room, I could instantly see she was in a lot of pain: she had great difficulty getting on the acupuncture couch, removing her outer garments or bending to take her shoes off. After the BM acupuncture treatment, she surprised herself (and me) when she got up from the couch, and put on her shoes and outer garments without the difficulties that she had had before.[1] She called me the next day to inform me that we had done better than 50 per cent – she had had at least an 80–90 per cent reduction in pain. Furthermore, she had had her first good night's sleep. She needed a few more treatments, and after the seventh BM acupuncture treatment I discharged her, essentially pain free.

Encouraged by these and other successes, I enrolled and studied with Dr Tan in New York and later in London. BM acupuncture is revolutionary and one of the key tools in my acupuncture toolbox for treating acute and chronic pain. It is so effective for most pain that it formed the basis of my PhD thesis. I often say to my patients that acupuncture is not magic but it could be magical, and is therefore invaluable for many of my patients who are so desperate for some level of pain relief.

FIVE ELEMENTS ACUPUNCTURE AND ALCHEMICAL HEALING
Moving Qi with needles and non-needling tools

A significant number of women with chronic pelvic pain also experience problems such as anxiety and depression that BM acupuncture is unlikely to help because it is very much a physical approach to pain. However, the psycho-emotional approach comes from the Five Elements acupuncture and Alchemical Healing that I've learned from Lorie Eve Dechar and incorporated into my clinical practice. 'Alchemy' is the 'art and science' of transformation, and I find this approach useful for patients who are interested in working with and transforming their emotional turmoil. Some of the skills that are used in Alchemical Healing include non-needling methods such as Inner Sensing, names of acupuncture points, Breathwork and Qi Gong that can move Qi and work synergistically with acupuncture to bring about positive changes in my patients. Qi is an ancient Chinese medicine concept that can be translated to mean our life force, without which there is no life.

Over many years, I also learned from my patients and other colleagues at cancer centres in New York City the importance of therapies such as Yoga, Reiki[2] and Meditation practice, as well as the primacy of connection, showing care, kindness and deep listening to ourselves and to our patients.

I recall a patient I treated using the Alchemical Healing approach that utilized non-needling tools many years ago. She was a middle-aged patient who had been hiccoughing non-stop for several days. She also had severe pain in the diaphragm area. All the relevant test results were within normal limits. She became very distressed and dehydrated because she had not been able to eat, drink or sleep. Prescribed medications for the pain and hiccoughing were not helping. With her body stooped over, she was pacing around the single room where she was being hydrated with an intravenous drip. She reminded me of a very fearful, distressed, anxious and restless animal caught in a cage. She could hardly complete a sentence without being interrupted by her hiccoughing. I invited her to listen to my voice and to place one of her hands over her heart area and another over the area between her belly button and pubic bone as she breathed in to a count of 5 and out to a count of 6, to feel the slow expansion and contraction of her chest and abdomen. I also held her heels with my hands, to ground and root the mind and Shen (spirit).[3] Gradually, her breathing slowed down, and became sonorous and rhythmic. She fell into a deep slumber. I left, returning two hours later to check in on her, and she was still fast asleep. She remained so by the time I left work at the end of the day. I learned that her hiccoughing had stopped, and she was no longer in pain. Equally important was that she had had the most restorative sleep ever. She was discharged the following morning.

Combining acupuncture with non-needling tools

Another patient came to me for acupuncture because of chronic pelvic pain that was no longer responding to medications. While surgery helped initially, the pain soon returned. She was in an extremely emotional state when I first met her. She was exhausted, as she had not had a good night's sleep for years. Her anxiety and depression made it very difficult for her to fall or stay asleep, which, in turn, made her fatigue and pain worse. When she was unable to fall asleep, her mind went through the same topics repeatedly, much like a dog chasing its own tail.

She described her anxiety as 'free-floating', that is, it was always there, but she could not pinpoint the exact cause of it. She also had an impending sense of doom. She attributed her depression to the stress and loss of her career, and thus the loss of her earning capability. Her life was often punctuated with panic attacks, which necessitated going to the Emergency Room as she thought she was having a heart attack. She had very dull eyes, and the spark that indicated the presence of the Shen was not there. The 'Shen' in Chinese medicine is loosely translated as our spirit, and in the Taoist tradition it is often represented as a small bird, the spirit animal of the Heart. This small bird flies away in the daytime and returns at night to nest in the Heart. In emotional or psychological turmoil, this small bird is unable to return home. When this happens, anxiety, a sense of unease and depression follow. What we needed to do was to coax the small bird back into the Heart space, so that peace and tranquillity could return to the woman's mind, body and spirit.

With one of her hands over the heart area and another over the lower dantian area, she followed my instructions to do the '5 breaths in and 6 breaths out' slow breathing before I started the acupuncture, and to continue throughout the treatment session. Once the needles had been inserted, I asked her to visualize an image of a small bird. I called this exercise 'Invitation to Return Home' (see Chapter 9). When she was ready, she could invite the small bird to return home to the Heart space. She was to observe without judgement if she could begin to feel a shift in her emotional state. This enabled her to access the innate self-healing capabilities that she already possessed within her. Often, I see a slow-down in the patient's breathing and pulse rate, and the return of colour to the face, which was exactly what happened to this patient. Further, at the end of our first session, even she noticed the difference in her eyes. She felt calmer. I gave her the written instructions for 'Invitation to Return Home', which she practised daily, and with great effect.

At the follow-up visit, her emotional state was much less chaotic. Her eyes lit up when she started to tell me how much the 'Invitation to Return Home' exercise had helped her deal with her anxiety and depression. Her pain had become more manageable, and she felt more optimistic as she now had the tool to deal with her sense of doom and any impending panic attack.

Although these examples feature patients with different pain conditions, the tools that are described here are equally useful for patients with most types of pain and who also suffer from anxiety and emotional and psychological distress. Medications did not work for my patient who had the hiccoughing and pain because she was very fearful, anxious and distressed. This patient and the patient with chronic pelvic pain needed some hands-on work, the comfort of touch and Breathwork, as well as the tools to access the body's ability to heal itself. All these worked effectively to soothe and calm their body, mind and spirit.

A PERSONAL JOURNEY

I now want to share a very personal story with you. Not so long ago, I went through a very challenging personal crisis. A very close and dear relative was diagnosed with a life-threatening disease. The anxiety and fear that welled up from deep inside me caused me to have panic attacks, fear, sleepless nights and a profound sense of dread. Over the months, with the help of Yoga, Meditation and Breathwork, I felt better, but the fear and sense of dread remained. I had several private sessions with my therapist/Alchemist Healer who gave me some Meditation work to steady my nervous system. Unfortunately, I continued to experience the fear and intense dread. This led to a discussion of my upbringing and childhood.

My therapist/Alchemist Healer helped me understand that these emotions most probably originated from my traumatic childhood experiences: my fear of being abandoned when my two brothers were born. She suggested that I enlarge a photograph of my little self and put it in a prominent place where I could love and reassure the little girl in me that my mother loved me and was not going to abandon me. This was accompanied by slow and easy Breathwork into my lower dantian (archaic energy; see Chapter 7), with some visualization of being safe and secure. As a reminder, the lower dantian is a source of our healing energies. I needed to own and befriend this fearful part of me that was probably buried deep in my unconscious and had intertwined itself into my nervous system to become part of myself. This daily practice shifted my fear and dread to an incredible sense of lightness and freedom. This transformation is the essence of Alchemical Healing.

My therapist/Alchemist Healer was Lorie Eve Dechar, another person who has had an enduring influence on my work. Lorie, and her husband Benjamin Fox, created Alchemical Healing, which cleverly weaves Chinese medicine (the Five Elements and Taoist philosophy) with Jungian archetypes, myths, Breathwork, dreamwork, active imagination, depth psychology (related to our conscious and unconscious) and body awareness to effect inner and outer changes. At the most profound level, Alchemical Healing is transformational in that it changes the way you feel, think, talk and respond to the events in your life and the world around you. For this to happen, you must recognize, want to and be prepared to do inner work, which is time consuming and difficult, although very much worth the effort. It is important that you work with an experienced and trained Alchemical Healer.

A NOTE ON TRIGGER POINTS

In working with women with chronic pelvic pain, I learned that trigger points can and do play a role in causing or contributing to the pain (see Chapter 5). When indicated, I deactivate trigger points and integrate this approach into my overall treatment for patients who have trigger points in the abdominal muscles or pelvic floor muscles. I feel extremely lucky that Dr Mark Seem (founder of the Tri-State Institute of Acupuncture, the school I attended) and Warner Seem made it their business to teach me how to palpate and deactivate trigger points, thus giving me a strong foundation in trigger point deactivation.

CONCLUDING THOUGHTS

When this book was first conceived, I had thought only of writing about BM acupuncture for chronic pelvic pain. As my writing evolved, it became clear that writing only about BM acupuncture would exclude a substantial part of my clinical work, that is, deactivating trigger points, the Alchemical Healing approach, and the non-needling tools and skills that synergistically work with acupuncture to help patients who are in pain, both physically and psychically. This combination of a physical and psycho-emotional approach to pain is not only restorative but also transformational. These are explained in subsequent chapters.

CHAPTER 2

CHRONIC PELVIC PAIN IN WOMEN

INTRODUCTION

In women, the pelvis is situated in the lower abdomen (the tummy from below the belly button), which contains organs such as the uterus (womb), ovaries, fallopian tubes, bladder and bowels. When the woman has pelvic pain, it usually involves one or more of these organs, muscles, nerves and blood vessels. If the woman has had intermittent or continuous pelvic pain for longer than three months, and it is bad enough to require treatment and it interferes with her daily living, by definition, this is chronic pelvic pain. These women are not alone, because it is estimated that one in seven women of childbearing age suffer from chronic pelvic pain, and that is a significant number of women.

CAUSES OF CHRONIC PELVIC PAIN

There are numerous potential causes of chronic pelvic pain. Many women have a cluster of symptoms that are related to conditions that include, but are not limited to, gynaecological diseases, such as endometriosis, adhesions due to pelvic inflammatory disease or surgery; gastrointestinal disease, such as irritable bowel syndrome (IBS); and genitourinary disease, such as painful bladder syndrome (PBS). (PBS used to be called interstitial cystitis, where there is pain and pressure in the bladder area.) Trigger points in the abdominal and pelvic floor muscles can also aggravate the pain (see Chapter 5 'Trigger Points). It is not unusual for a woman to present with a combination of endometriosis, PBS, trigger points and/or IBS.

In general, women with chronic pelvic pain seem to have a higher incidence of traumatic experiences such as a traumatic childhood and physical and/or sexual abuse. Approximately four out of ten women with chronic pelvic pain are found to have no apparent underlying cause(s) that can explain their pain (Howard 2000). Chronic pain with no underlying cause(s) is classified as primary chronic pain (Engeler *et al*. 2022). This inability to identify a reason for the pain generates further distress because it reinforces the misguided perception that their pain is not real. Nonetheless, whether they have underlying cause(s) or not, the pain experienced by this group of women is very real indeed, and in the not so recent past it has been too easily dismissed.

ENDOMETRIOSIS

'Endo what?' This is not an unusual response when it is the first time someone hears about endometriosis, which really speaks to the fact that many people have not heard of endometriosis, even though it is quite a common disorder. Because the chronic pain is caused by endometriosis, that is, with underlying cause(s), it is classified as secondary chronic pain.

Endometriosis is an oestrogen-dependent, neuro-inflammatory chronic condition where cells similar to those that line the uterus are found elsewhere in the body where they should not be, such as the lining of the wall of the pelvis (peritoneum), the ovaries, and the areas to the front, back and sides of the uterus, bladder and bowels. These endometrial-like growths are referred to as 'lesions' or 'implants', which behave like normal endometrial cells in that they react to hormones and have their monthly bleed, which results in pain, inflammation and scarring (Saunders and Horne 2021).

Pain is the most dominant symptom of endometriosis. While some women experience no or minimal symptoms, others have debilitating pain and fertility issues. About one in three women with endometriosis have difficulty getting pregnant, which is twice the rate of women without endometriosis (Prescott *et al.* 2016). Other common symptoms are pelvic pain, pain during and after sex, pain during bowel movement and urination, bloating, constipation and/or diarrhoea, and heavy menstruation as well as fatigue.

We do not yet know what causes endometriosis, although there are some theories, the most common one being the retrograde menstruation theory, which was first proposed by Dr John Sampson in the 1920s. This theory puts forward the idea that during a woman's monthly period, some menstrual blood and endometrial cells flow backward from the uterus via the fallopian tubes into the pelvis instead of flowing downward into the vagina and out (Horne and Saunders 2019).

Although the retrograde theory is quite widely accepted, it cannot explain the presence of endometrial cells in new-borns, males or young girls who have not started menstruating. It is believed that for some women, endometriosis is established soon after birth. This might explain why a certain number of female new-borns are observed to have vaginal bleeding that is caused by the womb shedding its lining, just like in menstruation, following the withdrawal of maternal ovarian hormones (Dekker *et al.* 2021).

How endometriosis is diagnosed

Most women with endometriosis start to have pelvic pain during adolescence. On average, most are not diagnosed until after consulting with several physicians, and therefore do not receive timely treatment (Ballard, Lowton and Wright 2006; Nnoaham *et al.* 2011). By the time they do receive the diagnosis, they will have been in pain for a significant number of years.

The gold standard for the diagnosis of endometriosis is a laparoscopy, when a biopsy is often obtained. The biopsied cells are examined under a microscope. A laparoscopy is keyhole surgery in which a small cut is made near the belly button where a laparoscope is inserted so that the surgeon can view the pelvic area projected on a television monitor.

Types of pelvic endometriosis

There are three types of pelvic endometriosis: superficial peritoneal endometriosis (SPE) (accounting for 80 per cent of endometriosis), deep endometriosis (DE) and ovarian endometriosis (endometrioma) (Horne and Saunders 2019). Among these three types, there appears to be no relationship between the pain levels and severity of the disease. Endometriosis lesions can also be found outside the pelvis, as far away as the upper abdominal organs, abdominal wall, diaphragm and the nervous system (Andres *et al.* 2020).

In SPE, the endometrial lesions are found on the peritoneum, a thin membrane that lines the abdomen and pelvis. These lesions look like little spots and can affect the pelvis extensively or minimally, and can co-exist with other subtypes of endometriosis. SPE can be difficult to treat surgically, especially if the disease is extensive.

In DE, the endometrial-like cells grow deeply (over 5mm) into where they are attached, such as the bowels, bladder, ureters or vagina, although there is no clear consensus as to its definition. DE is estimated to affect 20 per cent of women with pelvic endometriosis. The diagnosis of DE can be missed on a laparoscopy, but clinically suspected DE can be confirmed with a transvaginal ultrasound, and/ or magnetic resonance imaging (MRI). These technological advances offer an accurate method to diagnose DE because there is a poor relationship between severity of pain, its location and the subtype of endometriosis (Bazot and Daraï 2017).

Endometrioma are ovarian cysts containing old blood and lined by cells like endometrial tissue. Endometrioma is often referred to as 'chocolate cysts' because old blood looks like chocolate. Endometrioma also can cause adhesions and/or scarring to the nearby organs such as the bowels or pelvic side walls, leading to distortion of the pelvic structure as well as pain. The presence of endometrioma can be confirmed with a transvaginal ultrasound and/or MRI.

Types of endometriosis-associated pain

In my clinic I often come across patients with endometriosis who have a mix of inflammatory, nociceptive and/or neuropathic pain. Additionally, being subjected to chronic pain, patients can also experience a heightened sense of pain. This is called central sensitization, or amplification. Cross-organ sensitization occurs when pain from one organ with endometriosis spreads to nearby organ(s). Pain can also come from adhesions due to endometriosis or repeated surgery.

INFLAMMATORY, NOCICEPTIVE AND NEUROPATHIC PAIN
Inflammation is believed to play a key role in chronic pelvic pain. Inflammatory pain, as the name implies, is caused by chronic inflammation. In endometriosis the inflammation is fuelled by oestrogen in response to the endometrial-like tissue implants that often have their own blood and nerve supply. Patients describe inflammatory pain as dull, throbbing and constant (Carey, Till and As-Sanie 2017; Mu *et al.* 2018).

Closely related to inflammation is nociceptive pain. Inflammation triggers nociceptive pain by stimulating specialized nerve cells called nociceptors in the endometrium and endometriotic implants (Laux-Biehlmann, D'Hooghe and Zollner 2015). Nociceptive pain is typically experienced as sharp, aching or throbbing. A good example of nociceptive pain is when you have dental work or a cut on your finger. Neuropathic pain occurs when the nerve is damaged or irritated by the endometriosis lesions. Patients with neuropathic pain often complain of a shooting or burning pain as well as a tingling, pins-and-needles sensation.

In my clinical experience, I find that Balance Method (BM) acupuncture treatment is most effective for these types of pain.

CENTRAL SENSITIZATION OR AMPLIFICATION
As a result of chronic pain and a continuous pain signal being sent to the nervous system, some patients' pain can be amplified. This is like turning up the volume of a loudspeaker, except that it is the pain that

is being turned up. When this happens, typically the pain is felt all over the body, accompanied by fatigue, sleep disturbance and memory difficulties. These patients are very sensitive to touch and needling.

Central sensitization may be one of several explanations as to why, for some women, their pain persists even after surgery to remove the endometriosis lesions (As-Sanie *et al.* 2016; Brawn *et al.* 2014). This mechanism is also thought to underpin many chronic pain disorders such as irritable bowel syndrome (IBS) and chronic pelvic pain (Tracey 2016; Woolf 2011).

I see many patients with central sensitization in my 'pelvic pain' clinic. They are extremely sensitive to even gentle touch. Consequently, many cannot tolerate the insertion of acupuncture needles. Thus, treating these patients with acupuncture is very challenging and time consuming, but it is possible. I find that the patients can tolerate acupuncture treatment if it is approached with gentleness and the acupuncture needles are inserted very superficially, along the spine, on the Urinary Bladder meridian.

PAIN FROM CROSS-ORGAN SENSITIZATION

Cross-organ sensitization is when the pain from the endometriosis lesions spreads to nearby visceral organs such as the uterus, bowels and bladder. This is because these visceral organs in the pelvis, as well as other somatic structures (skin, bones, muscles and fascia), share the same nerve pathway, which makes it difficult to differentiate somatic from visceral pain (Schwartz and Gebhart 2014).

In reality, patients do not often present with clearly delineated pain types, or they may indeed have a combination of different pain types. Thus, it is sometimes difficult to know which type of pain is being treated. Pain from cross-organ sensitization is one such scenario.

PAIN FROM ADHESIONS

Adhesions are the result of inflammation that can be caused by endometriosis, surgery or pelvic inflammatory disease (Brill *et al.* 1995). They cause organs to stick together, leading to the distortion of the pelvic anatomy, pain and fertility problems. Adhesions have nerve fibres, which may explain why they cause pain, although sometimes the pain can be due to the ovary being trapped in the adhesions, cutting off the blood supply. Whether adhesions are rich in blood supply or not, transparent or dense, they are likely to play a major role in chronic pelvic pain (Thornton, Campeau and Dizerega 1997). However, the exact mechanism of why adhesions cause pain is not known.

Again, this makes it another very challenging condition to treat, from both a biomedicine and acupuncture perspective, especially when the adhesions are very severe.

IRRITABLE BOWEL SYNDROME, A GASTROINTESTINAL TRACT CONDITION

Many of my patients with chronic pelvic pain also suffer from IBS. They commonly present with abdominal discomfort with alternating loose stools and constipation, fatigue and back pain as well as dysmenorrhoea. Pain or discomfort is usually relieved by having a bowel movement. Women who suffer from IBS often experience depression and anxiety. IBS affects 10–20 per cent of the general population in developed countries, and is twice as common in women as in men. There is no cure for IBS and we do not know what causes it.

In my experience, I find that symptoms of IBS generally respond well to Chinese medicine therapies such as acupuncture, herbal medicine and moxibustion (the burning of dried herbs, e.g., mugwort (*Artemisia vulgaris*), placed in the appropriate acupuncture points to warm the interior).

Biomedicine treatment approach: lifestyle changes, diet and physical activities

The treatment approach outlined here is consistent with the National Institute for Health and Care Excellence (NICE)[4] guidelines on IBS (2008). The best clinical treatment approach centres on the individual patient and learning self-care skills such as dietary and lifestyle modifications. Dietary modifications include staying away from fizzy drinks and alcohol. It is also important that patients understand the difference between insoluble and soluble fibre so that they have an informed choice of what foods to include and exclude.

Insoluble fibre does not dissolve in water and digestive enzymes but gives bulk to the stool, which can make the IBS worse. Foods that are high in insoluble fibre are, for example, wheat bran and whole grains. Soluble fibre, on the other hand, retains water and turns gel-like during digestion, and is therefore kinder to the gut. Examples of foods that are high in soluble fibre are avocados, apples, blueberries, bananas, Brussels sprouts and carrots (Francis and Whorwell 1994). Further, to aid digestion it is important to eat regular meals and practise mindful eating to enhance the enjoyment and appreciation of the meal (see Chapter 9, 'Creating a Toolbox to Nurture and Nourish Ourselves'). It is best to work with a healthcare professional who has expertise in dietary management in order that the diet can be tailored to the needs and preferences of each patient.

Changes in lifestyle include regular participation in physical activity that suits the individual patient. There is data to suggest that physical activities such as Yoga may be beneficial to patients with IBS, although Yoga has not been specifically singled out as a recommendation by NICE (Kavuri *et al.* 2015) (for a further discussion on Yoga, see Chapter 9).

Medications

Antispasmodics such as peppermint oil may be effective in controlling the symptoms of IBS (Khanna, MacDonald and Levesque 2014). Depending on the individual patient, laxative or antimotility drugs to slow down gut movements may be recommended, and the dosage adjusted according to the patient's response. The aim is to maximize abdominal comfort and soften the stools to allow for an easy bowel movement.

For women who have depression and/or anxiety, antidepressants may be prescribed. For those patients who have not responded to other treatments, psychological intervention such as cognitive behavioural therapy and hypnotherapy may be considered (Ford *et al.* 2019).

For this group of patients who are willing and ready to do inner work, but who prefer not to take more medications, I find the Alchemical Healing approach invaluable.

PAINFUL BLADDER SYNDROME, A URINARY TRACT CONDITION

About two out of three women with chronic pelvic pain have painful bladder syndrome (PBS) (Tirlapur *et al.* 2013), and this statistic is reflected in my clinical experience. PBS affects more women than men. Most of my patients complain of pain and pressure in the bladder and pelvic area when the bladder is full, during urination, menstruation or sexual intercourse. Besides pain, they also experience an urgent and frequent need to urinate during the day and at night. Based on research from the American Urological Association (Hanno *et al.* 2015), PBS is described as 'an unpleasant sensation (pain, pressure, discomfort)' that is related to the urinary bladder, with urinary symptoms (such as sensations of pressure and discomfort that is related to the bladder filling, frequency, urgency in micturition) lasting more than six weeks, and no identifiable infection or cause.

Again, and frustratingly so, for both the patients and professionals, there is no known cause or cure for PBS, which makes it difficult to treat (Fall et al. 2010). It is thought that possible causes are infection, inflammation, damage to the bladder lining or the presence of trigger points in the pelvic floor muscles. The Royal College of Obstetricians & Gynaecologists briefly outlines some recommendations for managing PBS (RCOG 2016).

Biomedicine approach to managing PBS

As there is no cure for PBS, treatments are aimed at controlling symptoms by dietary modifications, stress management and analgesia for pelvic or bladder pain. Advice is tailored to each patient's preferences and responses to different treatments.

Dietary modifications

Because every patient is different, it is a matter of trial and error and using the food elimination method to find out what foods make a difference to the patient's pain. However, some studies suggest that certain foods, such as alcohol, coffee, citrus fruit, carbonated drinks, tea, chocolate and tomatoes, tend to make the pain worse (Warren *et al.* 2008). It is thus advisable for the patient to stop consuming these foods, or at least reduce their intake.

In my clinical work, I suggest to my patients to follow the food elimination method by keeping a diary. Very often, foods that aggravate pain in some women do not necessarily do so for others. Thus, it is important to individualize this approach, as one size does not fit all.

Stress management

Based on my clinical work, and reflected in some studies, teaching patients and emphasizing the important role of stress management techniques, such as conscious Breathwork with Meditation, listening to music, Yoga or regular physical activities, have been shown to help patients with PBS (O'Hare *et al.* 2013).

Medications

Pain medications such as paracetamol may help. Oral amitriptyline, a medication used for treating nerve pain, may be beneficial to control urinary urgency and frequency but has side effects such as a dry mouth, constipation, weight gain and blurred vision (Foster *et al.* 2010). Cimetidine, a medication used to treat stomach acid, is not licensed for the treatment of PBS, but it can be useful in controlling symptoms such as pain and needing to urinate at night (Thilagarajah, Witherow and Walker 2001).

Other options include the use of lidocaine, a local anaesthetic, to block nerves from sending pain messages to the bladder.

Neuromodulation may also be considered. If all else fails, referral to a multidisciplinary pain management team can be enacted. In many instances, that is when patients are referred to my clinic for acupuncture.

MYOFASCIAL PAIN SYNDROME
Myofascial pain syndrome is caused by trigger points that are exquisitely tender and knotty, with tight bands in the muscle and fascia. Trigger points in the abdominal muscles can cause pain in the stomach, sides and back, but they also refer pain to the organs in the abdomen and pelvic area. I often palpate for trigger points in the abdominal muscles, and when I find them, I deactivate them using acupuncture. When I suspect that triggers points are the cause of pelvic floor muscle pain, I usually advise the patient to see a physical therapist or physiotherapist if they are not seeing one already. This is because palpating and examining the pelvic floor is beyond my professional scope of practice as an acupuncturist. Women with trigger points in the pelvic floor muscles usually complain of pain during urination and sex, difficulty urinating, frequency or urgency in urination as well as constipation. (Trigger points that cause or contribute to chronic pelvic pain are covered in Chapter 5.)

Biomedicine management of myofascial pain syndrome
Treatment approaches will depend on the underlying cause(s) of the pain. Increasingly, there is a move towards putting patients at the centre of care because the 'old way' of doing business, where 'only the healthcare professional knows what's best for the patient', does not serve the patient and the professional well. Further, there is also an increased awareness that chronic pelvic pain is now understood to be a complex problem that is best managed by a multidisciplinary team with appropriate expert knowledge and skills, although it is not always possible to have a multidisciplinary team for various reasons, such as lack of money.

TREATMENT FOR ENDOMETRIOSIS-ASSOCIATED CHRONIC PELVIC PAIN

It is very important that women with endometriosis-associated pain understand what their pain management options are, and that they discuss their preference with their healthcare professionals. The different options available that are outlined here are consistent with the best practice approach recommended by NICE and the European Society of Human Reproduction and Embryology (ESHRE 2022).

Pain medications

For endometriosis-associated pelvic pain, paracetamol and/or non-steroidal anti-inflammatory drugs (NSAIDs) are often recommended, although there is no robust evidence for their effectiveness. It is also likely that women with chronic pelvic pain are already taking these medications, which can be bought over the counter. Like most drugs, there are risks involved with the frequent use of NSAIDs. These include inhibition of ovulation, headache, nausea, indigestion, dry mouth, gastric ulceration and increased bleeding (Bata *et al.* 2006). NSAIDs are thus not suitable for women who plan to get pregnant.

Hormonal suppression therapies

Hormonal suppression therapies include the combined oral contraceptive pill (COCP) (simply referred to as 'the pill'), progestogens (taken by mouth, injection or via an intra-uterine device) and gonadotropin-releasing hormone agonists (GnRHa; usually by injection). Most of these hormonal suppression therapies work by stopping or limiting the ovaries from producing oestrogen, and therefore reduce and/or stop the monthly bleed. The bleeding is known to create inflammation, scarring, adhesion (tissues sticking together) and pain. Remember that endometriosis needs oestrogen to develop and grow.

The pill is effective in reducing endometriosis-associated menstrual and non-menstrual pain as well as pain during sex. However, its side effects include nausea, headache, breast tenderness and low mood

(Vercellini *et al.* 1993). Progestogens can reduce endometriosis-associated pain, similar to the pill.

GnRHa reduces the body's production of oestrogen and testosterone (a male hormone, but women have a smaller amount of it). Although GnRHa is effective in reducing endometriosis-associated pain, its side effects can be quite severe. These include hot flushes, sleep difficulties, memory and bone loss. Because of its many serious side effects, GnRHa is usually reserved for women who have tried other treatment options unsuccessfully.

Neuromodulators

Neuromodulators are drugs that are promising in the management of chronic pain and endometriosis-associated pelvic pain. They are used for neuropathic pain. Most of them were originally prescribed for depression (e.g., amitriptyline,) and convulsion (e.g., gabapentin, pregabalin). Neuromodulators, as the name implies, reduce pain by modulating the central nervous system. The side effects of these drugs include weight gain, confusion, blurred vision and drowsiness. Therefore, not all women can tolerate them.

Surgery

When pain medications and hormonal therapies no longer work in controlling the pain, the key questions a woman with endometriosis-associated pain might ask is whether surgery will reduce or eliminate the pain, and what the side effects are. According to a review in 2009, surgery worked well to control the pain, but there was recurrence in 20 per cent of women at two years and 40–50 per cent at five years (Guo 2009). The aim of surgery is to remove as much of the endometriosis as possible by ablation (destroying the endometriosis by burning the implants using an electrical current) and/or excision (cutting out the endometriosis implants) as well as division of the adhesions.

Where endometriosis affects the bowels and bladder, a bowel surgeon (or colorectal surgeon) and/or urinary surgeon (or urologist) may have to be involved. Rarely, and depending on each woman's condition and preference, surgery to remove the uterus, ovaries and fallopian tubes may be undertaken. However, this approach may be considered for women who have not responded to conservative treatments, have completed their family or who do not wish to conceive (ESHRE 2022).

OTHER MODALITIES

In the UK, there is, however, a move towards including other therapies such as acupuncture, physiotherapy and cognitive therapy.

Acupuncture

In the scientific literature, the term 'acupuncture' is used to denote and is understood as the simple insertion of an acupuncture needle through the skin into selected points. Any practitioner who is traditionally trained in Chinese medicine will tell you that the insertion of an acupuncture needle is only one aspect of a complex and multifaceted acupuncture treatment. Recognizing this fact, this book covers in detail the needling (this chapter, as well as Chapters 3, 4 and 5) and non-needling components (Chapters 6 and 7) of acupuncture treatment. In this section, suffice to say that in 2021 the NICE committee considered that there was robust evidence to support the recommendation of acupuncture for chronic primary pain (pain with no apparent underlying cause). It was shown to reduce pain and improve the quality of life in the short term (up to three months) when compared with usual, standard biomedical care or sham (pretend) acupuncture.

The EXPPECT Centre for Pelvic Pain and Endometriosis at the Royal Infirmary of Edinburgh, where I currently work, is one of the few pelvic pain services in the UK that has a team of experts from different disciplines such as a consultant in pain medicine, a consultant gynaecologist, a clinical nurse specialist, a physiotherapist, a cognitive psychologist and a Chinese medicine practitioner (the author). As far as I know, it is the only centre in the UK to offer acupuncture for managing chronic pelvic pain in women. Interestingly, I believe that I am the only practitioner of Chinese medicine within the National Health Service (NHS) who provides not only acupuncture to manage the patient's physical pain, but also an emotional approach through the lens of the Five Elements theory and Alchemical Healing (see Chapters 6 and 7).

Physiotherapy

Pelvic physiotherapy has an important role for women who continue to experience pain in the bladder or bowels or during sexual intercourse despite optimal treatments. This may be due to a variety of reasons such as spasm or trigger points in areas such as the pelvic floor muscle and obturator internus muscle (found in the deep pelvic and gluteal area) or abdominal muscles.

Physiotherapy aims to release these trigger points, although this type of service may not be readily available in all healthcare settings.

Psychological approaches

Women with endometriosis-associated pain often report high levels of anxiety and depression, which can magnify their experience of pain, and can, in turn, affect their quality of life. It is therefore important that psychological approaches be made readily available, although their availability does vary across healthcare settings.

The aim of psychological approaches is to help women cope with the psychological impact of chronic pelvic pain. They must be tailored to the need of the individual and could take the form of a one-on-one consultation and/or a pain management programme, if available. This type of approach is very useful for enabling women to meet other women who are in the same 'boat', as well as to learn skills to pace themselves and adjust to and accept their condition (Lagana *et al.* 2017).

THE IMPACT OF LIVING WITH CHRONIC PELVIC PAIN

Chronic pelvic pain is a serious women's health issue because it affects a significant number of women of childbearing age. Further, chronic pelvic pain infiltrates into almost every aspect of a woman's life and seriously impacts on the quality of her life, as reflected in so many of my patients. This reminds me of a particular young lady whose life was turned upside down by endometriosis.

One day, many years ago, a young woman approached me after I had given a presentation at a conference on chronic pelvic pain and acupuncture. She had not been herself since her diagnosis of endometriosis many years before. She had tried surgical interventions, hormonal treatments and pain medications. None of these treatments had worked to relieve her pain. Medications had left her with many unpleasant side effects such as a dry mouth, constipation, brain fog and an inability to focus or fully function. Her medical condition had forced her into early retirement. She complained that she was no longer the capable and ambitious person that she used to be. Her life had been derailed. This young woman had lost her earnings, self-esteem and self-worth, and felt extremely socially isolated. Consequently, she nose-dived into a deep depression and her anxiety skyrocketed. Whatever little interest in sex she had had evaporated like mist on a hot day, never to return. All this proved too much and eventually led to her marital breakdown. She tried a session of acupuncture but discontinued because she was needle phobic. However, she continued her treatment because she had benefited from the various non-needling techniques such as learning self-care skills to manage her anxiety using Breathwork, and understanding the connection between telling herself a positive narrative and a sense of wellbeing. (Some of these techniques are discussed in Chapter 9.)

It is estimated that one in seven women of childbearing age are afflicted with chronic pelvic pain, but the real numbers could be much higher (Zondervan and Barlow 2000). Many women endure a complex set of pain in the genitals (vagina, labia), anus, perineum (sometimes aggravated by being seated), urethra, groin, sacrum, bowels, bladder, lower back, upper back and head (often reported as a headache or migraine). Some women are embarrassed to talk about it due to its very private nature. Like my young patient, many women experience anxiety, depression, fatigue and sleep disturbances that negatively impact on their quality of life, career and home as well as their overall health and wellbeing (Chong *et al.* 2018a). Many of the patients I treat suffer from these issues, and that is when I find the Alchemical Healing approach very useful, and sometimes transformative for the patients.

Sexual wellbeing and intimacy

Many women with chronic pelvic pain report a higher level of sexual dysfunction and dissatisfaction compared with women with no chronic pelvic pain (Tripoli *et al.* 2011). Sexual dysfunction is typically characterized by a significant disturbance to a woman's ability to respond sexually or experience sexual pleasure, causing distress to the woman as well as her partner. The anxiety and depression associated with chronic pelvic pain is most likely a contributing factor to sexual dysfunction. Besides the lack of desire, many women experience varying degrees of pain during and after intercourse. Some refrain from sexual activities, as the pain is so severe (Chong *et al.* 2018a). In a survey carried out in 2016, over 83 per cent of respondents who attempted sexual intercourse reported moderate to severe and 58 per cent high to very high painful sex, with its attendant feelings of guilt, rejection and frustration, which may end up in marital dysfunction or divorce, as was the case with the young patient mentioned here (Bryant *et al.* 2016). In an earlier study, 50 per cent of the 931 women with chronic pelvic pain who were surveyed reported that the pain had affected their relationship at some time during their life (de Graaff *et al.* 2013).

Work lives, loss of earnings and self-worth

Again, similar to the experience of my young patient, women who are diagnosed with chronic pelvic pain suffer from poor health. They have sleep disturbances (difficulty falling and staying asleep, as well as not feeling rested in the morning), fatigue and an inability to carry out their daily activities without pain medication. Their poor health and inability to participate in daily activities often means that they feel socially isolated. For some women, even holding a conversation poses a challenge because of fatigue, and some confided that they were beginning to lose friends. In the work arena, some women are unable to participate fully, leading to loss of working days, which eventually affects their earning capability. Some women were unable to cope with a full-time job and had to give up their career. They were unable to enjoy a 'normal' and personally fulfilling life that women without chronic pelvic pain can expect (Chong *et al.* 2018a; Simoens *et al.* 2011; Zondervan *et al.* 2001).

Personal and societal cost

With so many women of childbearing age who are affected, it is not surprising that chronic pelvic pain represents a huge economic burden on the individual as well as on the healthcare system. In the USA, according to a survey published in the *Journal of Obstetrics and Gynaecology Canada* in 2022, the total annual healthcare cost was estimated at over $2.8 billion, which roughly breaks down to between $1820 and $20,898 (including prescriptions, direct and indirect costs) per woman annually (Huang *et al.* 2021). In the UK, the annual healthcare costs were estimated at over $150 million in 1992 (Davies *et al.* 1992). Without a doubt, the financial burden in the UK must be much higher now.

CONCLUDING COMMENTS

Chronic pelvic pain is complex and challenging to treat and live with. It impacts negatively on the woman's quality of life as well as almost all aspects of her life. When surgery and/or drugs do not provide a satisfactory level of pain relief and/or have unpleasant and unwanted side effects, it is fair to say that there is very little left that biomedicine has to offer. It must be frustrating and frightening for those suffering from chronic pelvic pain. However, I would strongly advise that women with chronic pelvic pain start looking beyond drugs and surgery, especially if they do not have access to a multidisciplinary pain management team. They may want to consider other options such as acupuncture, psychological intervention or physiotherapy, with these integrated into conventional Western treatment. Equally important to a woman's overall management of her health is the question 'What else can I do for myself?' This is a very empowering question as it is likely to lead to a different path, one that will help women to enhance their ability to take care of themselves.

—— CHAPTER 3 ——

THE LOCAL BALANCE METHOD

INTRODUCTION

The results of the research I carried out for my PhD thesis suggest that the participants who received the Balance Method (BM) acupuncture treatment reported less pain, slept better and generally enjoyed a higher sense of wellbeing when compared with the two other groups that received NHS standard care or a traditional Chinese medicine health consultation (Chong *et al.* 2018a, 2018b). These results are preliminary; however, when taken together with my years of clinical experience, have convinced me that BM acupuncture has an important role in pain management. As I share this knowledge and skills with my fellow acupuncturists, prior knowledge of traditional Chinese medicine and the meridian system is assumed.

In BM acupuncture painful areas are not needled directly; instead, distal points are always selected to treat the pain. BM acupuncture has two primary components: Local Balance and Global Balance. Local Balance, as the name implies, is used to treat local symptoms such as pain, numbness and joint stiffness. Global Balance is the preferred approach for global problems, that is, when the pain is all over the body or pain that springs from the internal organs. I have used both Local and Global Balance for my patients with chronic pelvic pain as well as other related health issues, such as neck, shoulder and lower back pain or lower limb, muscle and joint pain as well as digestive issues. I do not want to overstate my claim, but over 95 per cent of the patients I treat experience immediate pain relief.

It is beyond the scope of this book to cover all the components of BM acupuncture. However, in this chapter I will focus on the Local Balance Method acupuncture, and in the next, on the Global Balance Method acupuncture. For those interested in learning more, I recommend you visit Dr Eileen Yue-Ling Han's website.[5]

Where necessary and appropriate, I have adapted some of the BM acupuncture treatment to suit my patients with chronic pelvic pain. However, I adhere to the late Dr Tan's teachings as closely as possible. A significant part of this chapter and the next is based on notes that I have gathered over the years as I attended Dr Tan's lecture series in both New York[6] and London.[7]

According to Dr Tan, BM acupuncture is effective in almost all painful conditions with a few exceptions, including pain due to significant anatomical or structural imbalance. In my patient population with chronic pelvic pain, this structural imbalance can be associated with extensive endometriosis-related adhesions (bands of scar tissue) where the internal organs (bowels, bladder, the reproductive system) are stuck together. This makes it a very challenging pain condition to treat.

In my clinical experience, treating this group of patients with BM acupuncture does not work very well. They report no pain during treatment, but once the needles are removed and they start moving and aggravating the bodily or anatomical structure, the pain returns almost immediately. However, for less severe adhesions or scar tissue, prolonged treatments are necessary to see an improvement.

Another condition where BM acupuncture is ineffective is psychic pain expressed as physical pain. For this group of patients, it is more appropriate to use the Five Elements acupuncture and Alchemical Healing approach (see Chapters 6 and 7).

BM acupuncture uses mostly Ashi points to treat pain, rather than textbook point location. In Chinese, 'shi' means 'yes', a response to the practitioner's palpation of a specific point in the body that is highly tender and sensitive; 'a' is an exclamation that is similar to 'Oh'; thus 'Ashi' is translated to mean 'Oh yes'.

Local and Global Balance are based on the same three-step algorithm.

THREE-STEP ALGORITHM

These three basic steps will help you to systematically pick the appropriate healthy meridian to treat the sick meridian and Ashi point(s) for treatment:

1. Identify the sick meridian: Ask the patient to point with one finger where they experience the most pain.

2. Identify the healthy meridian: Use one of the Five Systems (see Tables 3.1–3.5) to find the healthy meridian to balance the sick meridian.

3. Identify the Ashi point(s) on the healthy meridian for treatment: Use either the Mirror Method or Image Method.

LOCAL BALANCE USING THE FIVE SYSTEMS

The 12 meridians, or the Zang Fu (organs), do not function in isolation. In fact, the beauty and wonderment of it all is that they are intimately interconnected and related throughout our body. The Five Systems describe these connections and relationships among the 12 meridians as Yin–Yang, hand and foot relationships. Systems 1, 2 and 3 are derived from the Ba Gua (八卦) in the *Yi Ching* (*Book of Changes*) (see Tables 3.1, 3.2 and 3.3).[8] Systems 4 and 5 are based on the Chinese energy clock (see Tables 3.4 and 3.5).[9]

The simplest way to think about the Five Systems is to liken them to five different roadmaps to get to one destination. Using these roadmaps, you can systematically choose a healthy meridian to balance or treat the sick meridian. The Five Systems will make a lot of sense once you've familiarized yourself with the Chinese names of the meridians.

Table 3.1. System 1: Chinese meridian name sharing

Sick meridian	Needled meridian
Hand Tai Yin/LU	Foot Tai Yin/SP
Foot Tai Yin/SP	Hand Tai Yin/LU
Foot Yang Ming/ST	Hand Yang Ming/LI
Hand Yang Ming/LI	Foot Yang Ming/ST
Hand Shao Yin/HT	Foot Shao Yin/KI
Foot Shao Yin/KI	Hand Shao Yin/HT
Hand Tai Yang/SI	Foot Tai Yang/UB
Foot Tai Yang/UB	Hand Tai Yang/SI
Hand Jue Yin/PC	Foot Jue Yin/LR
Foot Jue Yin/LR	Hand Jue Yin/PC
Hand Shao Yang/TH	Foot Shao Yang/GB
Foot Shao Yang/GB	Hand Shao Yang/TH

Needle opposite side.
Meridian names: LU = Lung, LI = Large Intestine, ST = Stomach, SP = Spleen,
HT = Heart, SI = Small Intestine, KI = Kidney, UB = Urinary Bladder,
PC = Pericardium, LR = Liver, TH = Triple Heater, GB = Gall Bladder.

System 1 balances meridians that share the same name, for example hand Tai Yin/LU balances foot Tai Yin/SP (this name sharing system can be likened to a family surname). A hand meridian balances a foot meridian and vice versa. Yin meridians balance Yang meridians.

Hand ↔ foot and foot ↔ hand (balances ↔).

Table 3.2. System 2: Bie-Jing/Branching meridians

Sick meridian	Needled meridian
Hand Tai Yin/LU	Foot Tai Yang/UB
Foot Tai Yang/UB	Hand Tai Yin/LU
Hand Tai Yang/SI	Foot Tai Yin/SP
Foot Tai Yin/SP	Hand Tai Yang/SI
Hand Shao Yin/HT	Foot Shao Yang/GB
Foot Shao Yang/GB	Hand Shao Yin/HT

Hand Shao Yang/TH	Foot Shao Yin/KI
Foot Shao Yin/KI	Hand Shao Yang/TH
Hand Jue Yin/PC	Foot Yang Ming/ST
Foot Yang Ming/ST	Hand Jue Yin/PC
Foot Jue Yin/LR	Hand Yang Ming/LI
Hand Yang Ming/LI	Foot Jue Yin/LR

Needle either side.
Meridian names: LU = Lung, UB = Urinary Bladder, SI = Small Intestine, LI = Large Intestine, SP = Spleen, HT = Heart, GB = Gall Bladder, KI = Kidney, TH = Triple Heater, PC = Pericardium, ST = Stomach, LR = Liver.

System 2 balances opposite meridians such as hand Shao Yin/HT and foot Shao Yang/GB. Hand meridians are paired with foot meridians and foot meridians with hand meridians (the Shao Yin and Shao Yang pair is like a sister and brother relationship).

Hand ↔ foot and foot ↔ hand. Needle either side.

Table 3.3. System 3: Biao-Li/Interior–exterior pairs

Sick meridian	Needled meridian
Hand Tai Yin/LU	Hand Yang Ming/LI
Hand Yang Ming/LI	Hand Tai Yin/LU
Hand Shao Yin/HT	Hand Tai Yang/SI
Hand Tai Yang/SI	Hand Shao Yin/HT
Hand Jue Yin/PC	Hand Shao Yang/TH
Hand Shao Yang/TH	Hand Jue Yin/PC
Foot Tai Yin/SP	Foot Yang Ming/ST
Foot Yang Ming/ST	Foot Tai Yin/SP
Foot Shao Yin/KI	Foot Tai Yang/UB
Foot Tai Yang/UB	Foot Shao Yin/KI
Foot Jue Yin/LR	Foot Shao Yang/GB
Foot Shao Yang/GB	Foot Jue Yin/LR

Needle opposite side.

Meridian names: LU = Lung, LI = Large Intestine, HT = Heart, SI = Small Intestine, PC = Pericardium, TH = Triple Heater, SP = Spleen, ST = Stomach, KI = Kidney, UB = Urinary Bladder, LR = Liver, GB = Gall Bladder.

System 3 balances the interior–exterior (Biao-Li), which has a Zang Fu (organ) relationship, such as hand Tai Yin/LU and hand Yang Ming/ LI and vice versa. This is the only system that balances hand meridians with hand meridians and foot meridians with foot meridians (I like to remember this as my relationship with my cousin).

Hand ↔ hand and foot ↔ foot. Needle the opposite side.

Table 3.4. System 4: Chinese clock opposites

Sick meridian	Needled meridian
Hand Tai Yin/LU	Foot Tai Yang/UB
Hand Yang Ming/LI	Foot Shao Yin/KI
Foot Yang Ming/ST	Hand Jue Yin/PC
Foot Tai Yin/SP	Hand Shao Yang/TH
Hand Shao Yin/HT	Foot Shao Yang/GB
Hand Tai Yang/SI	Foot Jue Yin/LR
Foot Tai Yang/UB	Hand Tai Yin/LU
Foot Shao Yin/KI	Hand Yang Ming/LI
Hand Jue Yin/PC	Foot Yang Ming/ST
Hand Shao Yang/TH	Foot Tai Yin/SP
Foot Shao Yang/GB	Hand Shao Yin/HT
Foot Jue Yin/LR	Hand Tai Yang/SI

Needle either side.

Meridian names: LU = Lung, UB = Urinary Bladder, LI = Large Intestine, KI = Kidney, ST = Stomach, PC = Pericardium, SP = Spleen, TH = Triple Heater, HT = Heart, GB = Gall Bladder, SI = Small Intestine, LR = Liver.

System 4 balances meridians on the Chinese clock such as foot Yang

Ming/ST and hand Jue Yin/PC (I like to remember this as my opposite neighbour).

Hand ↔ foot and foot ↔ hand. Needle either side.

Table 3.5. System 5: Chinese clock neighbours

Sick meridian	Needled meridian
Hand Tai Yin/LU	Foot Jue Yin/LR
Hand Yang Ming/LI	Foot Yang Ming/ST
Foot Yang Ming/ST	Hand Yang Ming/LI
Foot Tai Yin/SP	Hand Shao Yin/HT
Hand Shao Yin/HT	Foot Tai Yin/SP
Hand Tai Yang/SI	Foot Tai Yang/UB
Foot Tai Yang/UB	Hand Tai Yang/SI
Foot Shao Yin/KI	Hand Jue Yin/PC
Hand Jue Yin/PC	Foot Shao Yin/KI
Hand Shao Yang/TH	Foot Shao Yang/GB
Foot Shao Yang/GB	Hand Shao Yang/TH
Foot Jue Yin/LR	Hand Tai Yin/LU

Needle opposite side.
Meridian names: LU = Lung, LR = Liver, LI = Large Intestine, ST = Stomach, SP = Spleen, HT = Heart, SI = Small Intestine, UB = Urinary Bladder, KI = Kidney, PC = Pericardium, TH = Triple Heater, GB = Gall Bladder.

System 5 balances immediate neighbours on the Chinese clock such as hand Yang Ming/LI and foot Yang Ming/ST (I like to remember this as my nextdoor neighbour).

Hand ↔ foot and foot ↔ hand. Needle the opposite side.

There is, of course, System 6, which can be used to treat its own meridian and is not shown here.

MIRROR AND IMAGE METHODS FOR POINT SELECTION

The focus for now is on the Mirror and Image Methods, which are two of the several methods for point selection.

The Mirror Method

The Mirror Method (see Table 3.6) maps the reflex between limbs and locates the specific area of the limb to be treated. This means, for example, that pain in the elbow is reflected in the knee, the area to be treated. Therefore, the knee balances the elbow and vice versa. In the Reverse Mirror Method, the shoulder mirrors the ankle and vice versa.

Those of you who are not acupuncturists can still use the Mirror and Image Methods to locate the area of treatment. Instead of using acupuncture needles, simply apply acupressure or gently massage the identified area(s).

Table 3.6. The Mirror Method

↔ Balances	
Mirror Method	**Reverse Mirror Method**
Shoulder ↔ Hip	Shoulder ↔ Ankle
Upper arm ↔ Thigh	Upper arm ↔ Lower leg
Elbow ↔ Knee	Elbow ↔ Knee
Forearm ↔ Lower leg	Forearm ↔ Thigh
Wrist ↔ Ankle	Wrist ↔ Hip joint
Hand ↔ Foot	Hand ↔ Hip
Fingers ↔ Toes	Fingers ↔ Top of hip

The Image Method

The Image Method (see Table 3.7) provides another way of selecting the specific area of the limbs, head or trunk for treatment. While the Mirror Method balances limb with limb, the Image Method balances the limbs/hands with the head/trunk of the body and vice versa. The corresponding area to be needled often feels tender and tight (Ashi points).

The Reverse Image Method is obtained by inverting the images. For example, if the testicles or anus is the affected area, the finger is needled using the Image Method, and the top of the head is needled using the Reverse Image Method.

Table 3.7. The Image Method

To be needled	Image Method (affected area)	Reverse Image Method (affected area)
Finger/Toe	Testicles, external genitalia (women), anus	Top of head
Hand/Foot	Genitals, coccyx, sacrum	Head, base of skull
Wrist/Ankle	Bladder, lumbosacral area	Neck, neck joint
Forearm/Lower leg	Lower abdomen, lower back	Upper abdomen, rib cage, mid-upper back
Elbow/Knee	Umbilicus level, lumbar 2, waist	Umbilicus level, lumbar 2, waist
Upper arm/Upper leg	Upper abdomen, rib cage, chest, mid-upper back	Lower abdomen, lower back
Shoulder/Hip joint	Neck, jaw, base of skull	Sacrum, genitals, coccyx

THE FIVE SYSTEMS AND CASE STUDIES

Balancing system 1: Chinese meridian name sharing

Besides sharing the same Chinese meridian name, System 1 is based on the anatomical relationships of the limbs and the six meridians (see Table 3.1). In System 1, a hand Yin meridian balances a foot Yin meridian, and a hand Yang meridian balances a foot Yang meridian. I use two case studies here to illustrate the basic three-step algorithm, the Five Systems and the Mirror and Image Methods.

CASE STUDY 1: MIRROR METHOD

This patient complains of pain in the right elbow, at LI 11:

1. Diagnose the sick meridian(s): Ask the patient to point with one finger the location of most pain – the hand Yang Ming/ LI (right).

2. Find the healthy meridian(s) to balance the sick meridian(s): Foot Yang Ming/ST.

3. Find the Ashi point(s) on the foot Yang Ming/ST meridian (left): Use the Mirror Method (see Table 3.6) as limb balances limb. Palpate the foot Yang Ming/ST meridian on the lower leg (left), around the left knee (ST 36 area) for Ashi point(s) (the elbow mirrors the knee). Needle the most tender and sensitive point(s) as reported by the patient.

CASE STUDY 2: IMAGE METHOD

This patient complains of endometriosis-associated pain on the right side of the lower abdomen:

1. Diagnose the sick meridian(s): Ask the patient to point with one finger the location of most pain – ST 26 area – the foot Yang Ming/ST (right).

2. Find the healthy meridian(s) to balance the sick meridian(s): Hand Yang Ming/LI.

3. Find the Ashi point(s) on the hand Yang Ming/LI meridian (left): Use the Reverse Image Method (see Table 3.7) as the limb balances the torso/head and vice versa. Palpate the hand Yang Ming/LI on the forearm for Ashi point(s) (the upper arm reverse images the lower abdomen). Needle the Ashi point(s) around LI 10 and LI 11.

Balancing system 2: Bie Jing/branching meridians

System 2 balances the Yin–Yang branching meridians of the hands and feet (see Table 3.2). The Yin meridians of the hand balance the Yang meridians of the foot, and the Yin meridians of the foot balance the Yang meridians of the hand.

CASE STUDY 1: MIRROR METHOD

The same patient with pain in the right elbow, around LI 11:

THE LOCAL BALANCE METHOD

1. Diagnose the sick meridian(s): Ask the patient to point with one finger the location of most pain – the hand Yang Ming/LI (right).

2. Find the healthy meridian(s) to balance the sick meridian: Foot Jue Yin/LR.

3. Find the Ashi point on the foot Jue Yin/LR meridian (either side): Use the Mirror Method to select the area of the limb to be treated. Palpate the foot Jue Yin/LR meridian on the lower leg for Ashi point(s) (the elbow mirrors the knee). Needle the Ashi point(s), around LR 8.

CASE STUDY 2: IMAGE METHOD

The same patient who complains of endometriosis-associated pain on the right side of the lower abdomen:

1. Diagnose the sick meridian(s): Ask the patient to point with one finger the location of most pain – ST 26 area, foot Yang Ming/ST (right).

2. Find the healthy meridian(s) to balance the sick meridian: Hand Jue Yin/PC.

3. Find the Ashi point(s) on the hand Jue Yin/PC meridian (below PC 3): Use the Image Method to select the area of the limb to be treated. Palpate the hand Jue Yin/PC meridian on the forearm for Ashi point(s). Needle either side.

Balancing system 3: Biao-Li/interior–exterior pairs

System 3 employs the Zang Fu (organs) interior–exterior relationships (see Table 3.3). This system balances the hand meridians with the hand meridians and the foot meridians with the foot meridians, using the Yin–Yang pair. According to Dr Tan, System 3 is usually the best for injury and trauma, although in clinical practice it is important to also be guided by the idea of treating a similar anatomical structure.

CASE STUDY 1: MIRROR METHOD

The same patient with pain on the outside of the right elbow, around LI 11:

1. Diagnose the sick meridian(s): Ask the patient to point with one finger the location of most pain – hand Yang Ming/LI (right).

2. Find the healthy meridian(s) to balance the sick meridian(s): Hand Tai Yin/LU (left).

3. Find the Ashi point(s) on the hand Tai Yin/LU meridian: Use the Mirror Method to select the area of the limb for treatment. Palpate and needle around LU 5 (left) for Ashi points.

CASE STUDY 2: IMAGE METHOD

The same patient who complains of endometriosis-associated pain on the right side of the lower abdomen:

1. Diagnose the sick meridian(s): Ask the patient to point with one finger the location of most pain – ST 26 area, foot Yang Ming/ST (right).

2. Find the healthy meridian(s) to balance the sick meridian(s): Foot Tai Yin/SP.

3. Find the Ashi point(s) on the foot Tai Yin/SP meridian (left): Use the Image Method to find the area for treatment. Palpate the foot Tai Yin/SP (around SP 8 or SP 9 on the lower leg for Ashi point(s). Needle the most sensitive Ashi point(s).

Balancing system 4: Chinese Qi (energy) clock opposites

Figure 3.1 shows the Chinese Qi (energy) clock (see also Table 3.4). It takes 24 hours for the flow of Qi to complete its 12-meridian cycle.

THE LOCAL BALANCE METHOD

Every two-hour interval is related to a specific meridian. Each meridian has a peak two-hour Qi flow, and its counterpart, which is on the opposite side of the clock, has its lowest. For example, the peak two-hour Qi flow for the foot Yang Ming/ST meridian is between 7am and 9am, and its counterpart, the hand Jue Yin/PC Qi flow, is at its lowest. System 4 makes use of this idea and the notion that the opposite meridians balance each other. A Yang meridian balances a Yin meridian and vice versa. The hand balances the foot and the foot the hand. Thus, hand Shao Yin/HT balances foot Shao Yang/GB; foot Yang Ming/ST balances hand Jue Yin/PC and so on. You will have noticed that System 4 is the same as System 2. Needle on the same or opposite side.

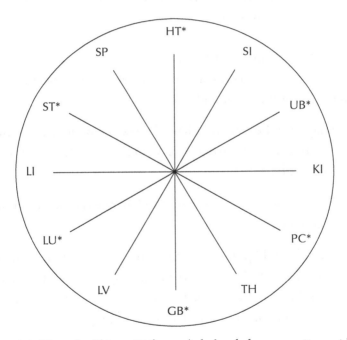

Figure 3.1. Using the Chinese Qi (energy) clock to balance opposite meridians: Yin balances Yang and vice versa; hand balances foot and vice versa

CASE STUDY 1: MIRROR METHOD

Using the patient who complains of pain in the right elbow around LI 11:

1. Diagnose the sick meridian(s): Ask the patient to point with one finger the location of most pain – hand Yang Ming/LI (right).

2. Find the healthy meridian(s) to balance the sick meridian(s): Foot Shao Yin/KI (left).

3. Find the Ashi point(s) on the foot Shao Yin/KI meridian: Use the Mirror Method to select the area of the limb for treatment. Palpate around LR 8 area for Ashi point(s). Needle the most sensitive Ashi point(s).

CASE STUDY 2: IMAGE METHOD

The same patient who complains of endometriosis-associated pain on the right side of the lower abdomen:

1. Diagnose the sick meridian(s): Ask the patient to point with one finger the location of most pain – ST 26 area, foot Yang Ming/ST (right).

2. Find the healthy meridian(s) to balance the sick meridian(s): Hand Jue Yin/PC.

3. Find the Ashi point(s) on the hand Jue Yin/PC meridian: Use the Image Method to find the area for treatment. Palpate the hand Jue Yin/PC on the forearm for Ashi point(s) (below PC 3). Needle the most sensitive Ashi point(s).

Balancing system 5: Chinese Qi clock neighbours

In System 5, neighbouring meridians that share the same name balance each other (see Figure 3.2 and Table 3.5). For example, hand Yang Ming/LI balances foot Yang Ming/ST and hand Shao Yang/TH balances foot Shao Yang/GB. System 5 is like System 1.

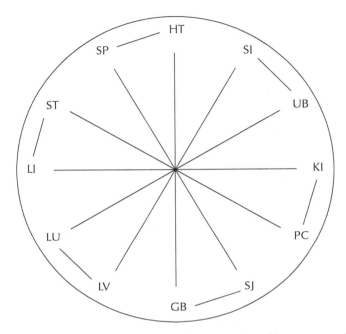

Figure 3.2. System 5: Balancing name sharing and neighbouring meridians

CASE STUDY 1: MIRROR METHOD

The same patient with the pain in the right elbow around LI 11:

1. Diagnose the sick meridian(s): Ask the patient to point with one finger the location of most pain – hand Yang Ming/LI (right).

2. Find the healthy meridian(s) to balance the sick meridian(s): Foot Yang Ming/ST (left).

3. Find the Ashi point(s) on the foot Yang Ming/ST meridian: Use the Mirror Method to select the Ashi point(s) for treatment. Palpate around ST 36 for Ashi point(s). Needle the most sensitive point(s).

CASE STUDY 2: IMAGE METHOD

The same patient who complains of endometriosis-associated pain on the right side of the lower abdomen:

1. Diagnose the sick meridian(s): Ask the patient to point with one finger the location of most pain – ST 26 area, foot Yang Ming/ST (right).

2. Find the healthy meridian(s) to balance the sick meridian(s): Hand Yang Ming/LI.

3. Find the Ashi point(s) on the hand Yang Ming/LI meridian: Use the Image Method to find the area for treatment. Palpate the hand Yang Ming/LI on the forearm for Ashi point(s) (around LI 10, LI 11). Needle the most sensitive Ashi point(s).

Note: In System 6, use the same meridian to treat itself. For example, hand Tai Yin/LU can treat hand Tai Yin/LU and so on.

IN-DEPTH CASE STUDY: TREATING CHRONIC PELVIC PAIN USING THE IMAGE METHOD

This young patient had had endometriosis-associated chronic pelvic pain for about 15 years, and was no longer able to obtain satisfactory pain relief from conventional medicine approaches. She was careful in the use of the stronger opioid drugs because of the side effects and the likelihood of dependency or addiction. The pain that she described as sharp and stabbing was focused on the right lower abdomen with a scale of 9–10 out of 10 (10 being most painful). At worst, she had to take to her bed and could not go to work. On better days, the pain could be a dull throb. She was never without pain. It was a matter of how serious the pain was and how much it interfered with her life. Gentle movement made the pain better, but house-cleaning activities such as vacuuming made it worse. Her pain responded to heat most of the time.

Following the BM acupuncture three-step algorithm:

1. Identify the sick meridian: At this very important meridian(s) diagnostic step, the patient was instructed to point with one finger where the most pain was: around GB 27 and GB 28 on the right side. The sick meridian was the foot Shao Yang/GB.

2. Identify the healthy meridian: From the Five Systems (see Tables 3.1–3.5), the choice is among:

   a. Hand Shao Yang/TH (Systems 1 and 5).

   b. Hand Shao Yin/HT (Systems 2 and 4).

   c. Foot Jue Yin/LR (System 3).

   Foot Jue Yin/LR was the meridian of choice. This was primarily based on palpating all three meridians and their Ashi points to explore which meridian to choose based on the patient's feedback. This is a very important part of the learning process and in building your clinical skills as well as your confidence. As you become more experienced, you will know intuitively the most appropriate meridian to choose.

3. Identify the Ashi point(s) on the foot Jue Yin/LR meridian: The Image Method was used, as the lower leg balances the lower abdomen. Palpation was done on foot Jue Yin/LR on the lower leg for Ashi points. Needles were inserted into the most sensitive Ashi points bilaterally around the Ashi points of LR 7 and LR 8. The patient reported a significant drop in pain level almost as soon as the needles were inserted. The needles were left in for at least 40 minutes, although Dr Tan's advice was to leave the needles for longer.

The beauty of BM acupuncture is that if it is done correctly, it gives immediate pain relief. This patient reported a satisfactory reduction in pain of over 70 per cent. She continued with the BM acupuncture treatment once a week, which kept her pain under control.

MATRIX ANALYSIS: PELVIC PAIN THAT INVOLVES MULTIPLE MERIDIANS

Many of my patients' pain patterns do not always fall neatly into one or even two meridian(s). This is because they have a complex pain pattern that involves multiple meridians and in areas that have no established acupuncture points/meridians. Furthermore, they often report pain in their bowels, bladder, groin, shoulders, lower back, lower limbs, muscles and joints. This complex pain pattern is very challenging to manage. In this section, I will showcase how to treat women with complex pain, which involves several meridians.

Case study 1

This 29-year-old patient complained of endometriosis-associated pelvic pain for many years. Her chief complaint was sharp and stabbing pain across the entire lower abdomen (she described her pain as above 10, 10 being the most painful). She was taking several pain medications, but had not achieved satisfactory pain relief. At times the pain was so bad that she almost fainted.

BM ACUPUNCTURE THREE-STEP ALGORITHM

1. Identify the sick meridians: With one finger, the patient pointed across her entire lower abdomen, which involved the following meridians: foot Yang Ming/ST, foot Tai Yin/SP, foot Shao Yang/GB and foot Shao Yin/KI.

2. The healthy meridians to balance the sick meridians were:

    a. Hand Shao Yang/TH and hand Shao Yin/HT balance the three sick meridians: SP, GB and KI (see the last three rows from the bottom up in Table 3.8).

    b. The second choice is hand Yang Ming/LI and hand Jue Yin/PC because they balance the two sick meridians: ST and KI.

THE LOCAL BALANCE METHOD

Table 3.8. Matrix analysis: choice of meridians
(indicated with *) to balance the sick meridians

	System 1	System 2	System 3	System 4	System 5
Sick meridians	Healthy meridians	Healthy meridians	Healthy meridians	Healthy meridians	Healthy meridians
ST	LI	PC	SP	PC	LI
SP	LU	SI	ST	TH*	HT*
GB	TH*	HT*	LR	HT*	TH*
KI	HT*	TH*	UB	LI	PC

Note: The smart choice is (a) since HT and TH balance SP, GB and KI. That, however, leaves the ST meridian not addressed. LI can always be added to balance the ST meridian if necessary.

3. In the Image Method, the forearm balances the lower abdomen and lower back. Thus palpation along hand Shao Yang/TH and hand Shao Yin/HT were undertaken bilaterally on the forearm to look for Ashi point(s), that is, the most tender and sensitive points, which was around TH 5. The needles were inserted into the Ashi point bilaterally in the direction and depth of the palpation. The pain was reduced by 50 per cent.

   Next, hand Shao Yang/HT was palpated bilaterally. The most sensitive Ashi point was around the HT 3 area. Needles were inserted bilaterally in the direction and depth of palpation. The patient reported that she was almost pain free after the needles were inserted. The needles were stimulated manually and removed after 30–40 minutes, or longer, if time allowed.

The patient continued to receive BM acupuncture once a week (although it would have been ideal if she could have received her treatments at least twice per week) until her chronic pelvic pain was satisfactorily controlled. Her appointments were tapered to once every two weeks, and then with a follow-up appointment once a month. Patients with endometriosis-associated pelvic pain tend to have flare-ups, a sudden increase in pain, making the trajectory difficult to predict. Thus, she was advised to call for an appointment or to see her gynaecologist should that happen.

Case study 2

1. Identify the sick meridians: In the next treatment, the same patient identified the sick meridians as: ST, SP, KI and LR (see Table 3.9).

Table 3.9. Choice of meridians (indicated with *) to balance the sick meridians

	System 1	System 2	System 3	System 4	System 5
Sick meridians	Healthy meridians	Healthy meridians	Healthy meridians	Healthy meridians	Healthy meridians
ST	LI*	PC*	SP	PC*	LI*
SP	LU	SI	ST	TH	HT
KI	HT	TH	UB	LI*	PC*
LR	PC*	LI*	GB	SI	LU

2. Identify the healthy meridian: From the above matrix:

    a. LI balances three sick meridians ST, KI, LR (see the 1st, 2nd and 4th row from the bottom up).

    b. PC balances the same three sick meridians ST, KI, LR (1st, 2nd and 4th row from the bottom up). We now need to identify a healthy meridian to balance the SP meridian:

    c. TH balances SP, KI.

    d. HT balances SP, KI.

    e. LU balances SP, LR.

    f. SI balances SP, LR.

We can choose to combine LI with one of the meridians from (c) to (f): LI and TH (a combination of (a) and (c)), which allows us to treat all the sick meridians of ST, KI, LR and SP, *or* LI and HT (a combination of (a) and (d)), which allows us to treat all the sick meridians: ST, KI, LR and SP, *or* LI and LU (a combination of (a) and (e)), which allows us to treat all the sick meridians: ST, KI, LR and SP, *or* LI and SI (a combination of (a) and (f)), which allows us to treat all the sick meridians: ST, KI, LR and SP.

The second choice is to combine PC with one of the meridians from (c) to (f): PC and TH, *or* PC and HT, *or* PC and LU, *or* PC and SI.

3. By doing the matrix analysis, we need only to needle two points to balance all four sick meridians. The next step is to select the Ashi points for needling using the Image Method.

4. Identify the Ashi point(s): Following the Image Method, palpation of the TH and LI meridians was undertaken bilaterally on the forearm to look for Ashi point(s), that is, the most tender and sensitive points: around TH 5 and LI 4. The needles were inserted into the Ashi point bilaterally in the direction and depth of the palpation with significant pain relief.

These two case studies underline the usefulness of matrix analysis in the real world of clinical practice. Matrix analysis looks complicated, but if you follow the steps slowly, patiently and carefully, you will get it, eventually.

CONCLUDING THOUGHTS

As I come to the end of this chapter, I want to give a word of encouragement to the acupuncturists who are new to BM acupuncture. If you follow the steps outlined in this chapter, you, and equally important, your patients, will be happy with the result. The pain relief, sleep improvement and general sense of wellbeing that my patients achieved mirror the preliminary findings in my PhD study.

As I alluded to earlier, our patients do not come with pain patterns that fall neatly on to one meridian and acupuncture point. Some have very complex condition(s) where too many sick meridians are involved. When this happens, I find using Dr Tan's Global Balance Method very helpful. I will introduce Global Balance in the next chapter. In addition, many patients come with other psycho-emotional-spiritual problems. This is when I integrate the approach of Alchemical Healing into my clinical practice once the physical pain has been addressed, or sometimes these are addressed almost simultaneously.

I would like to conclude this chapter with some clinical pearls that I hope will be helpful. These are small but fundamentally important steps we must pay attention to if we want to have success in reducing our patients' pain.

CLINICAL PEARLS

- *Anatomical similarity:* Be guided also by anatomical similarity when choosing the meridians to treat. For instance, treat muscle with muscle, tendon with tendon and bone with bone.

- *Specific needling instructions:* For best results, always needle the selected Ashi points based on the direction and depth of your palpation to achieve optimum pain relief. Inattention to these very important details will result in disappointment.

- *Always get feedback from the patient:* Do not ask the patient if they have any pain; ask them where their pain is after the needles have been inserted. This is because when the worst pain has been taken care of, the next layer of pain located in another part of the body starts to surface. If your patient reports no pain relief, repeat the BM acupuncture three-step algorithm to treat the pain until satisfactory pain relief is achieved.

- *Listen carefully and pay attention to what the patient is telling you or not telling you!* By listening between the spaces and silence as well as looking at the patient's facial expressions and body language, you gain information about the patient that you may otherwise have missed.

- *How many times per week should we ensure the patient gets treatment?* I am frequently asked how often the patient should receive treatment. Well, the answer is – it depends. A patient with very severe chronic pelvic pain will probably need more frequent treatment than another with less severe pain. It also depends on other constraints such as time and the patient's financial situation. In my experience, the best approach is to discuss with the patient the best possible treatment plan based on these factors.

— CHAPTER 4 —

THE GLOBAL BALANCE METHOD

INTRODUCTION

In Chapter 3 I presented the Local Balance Method, which is used to treat local symptoms such as pain, numbness or joint stiffness, as well as the Image and Mirror Methods for point selection. The Global Balance Method presented in this chapter is indicated in multiple problems that involve many meridians such as chronic pelvic pain, irritable bowel syndrome (IBS), fibromyalgia, headaches and backache. In this chapter I will also introduce the meridian conversion method for point selection, which is illustrated with two examples. It is important to note that in the Global Balance Method, one of two conditions – Static Balance and Dynamic Balance – must be satisfied. Although it is beyond the scope of this chapter to cover the many patterns that can evolve from the Global Balance Method, I have included Dr Tan's Eight and Twelve Magical Points (Tan 2003). I find the Twelve Magical Points particularly useful, and thus use it frequently to address complex health problems such as fibromyalgia, IBS, painful bladder syndrome (PBS), stress-related problems and hormonal imbalance.

STATIC BALANCE
Structures, lines and meridians

In Static Balance, 'static', as the name implies, has no movement. Conceptually, however, it provides stability to a structure, as is necessary in a building, for example. This contrasts with Dynamic Balance, where 'dynamic' reflects the constant flux of the movement of Qi as seen, for instance, in the changing of the seasons and day to night to day to night. To explain how Global Balance works, Dr Tan borrowed four engineering structures or symbols – A, B, C and D (see Figure 4.1).

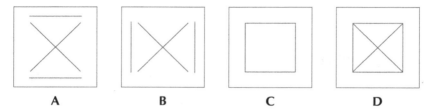

Figure 4.1. Four structures of Static Balance that represent the relationships among the meridians in any pattern

The four structures, A, B, C and D, are made up of vertical, horizontal and diagonal lines. They describe the relationships among the meridians in any of the Five Systems:

- Diagonal lines are associated with Systems 1 and 5
- Vertical lines are associated with Systems 2 and 4
- Horizontal lines are associated with System 3.

STRUCTURE A

Figure 4.2 shows that in Structure A, the horizontal lines connect Segments I to II and III to IV, and the diagonal lines connect Segments I to III and II to IV. The lines that connect each segment balance each other in the Five Systems of Balance Method (BM) acupuncture. In other words, the meridians that are selected for treatment must satisfy structure A:

THE GLOBAL BALANCE METHOD

- Segment I balances Segment II (System 3)
- Segment III balances Segment IV (System 3)
- Segment I balances Segment III (System 1)
- Segment II balances Segment IV (System 1).

Note that there are no lines connecting Segments I to IV and Segments II to III, which means they cannot be used to balance each other, based on the Five Systems.

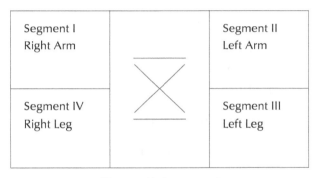

Figure 4.2. Structure A

STRUCTURE B

Figure 4.3 shows that in Structure B, the vertical lines connect Segments I to IV and II to III. The diagonal lines connect Segments 1 to III and II to IV. As in Structure A, the meridians selected for treatment must satisfy Structure B in the Five Systems:

- Segment I balances Segment IV (Systems 2 and 4)
- Segment II balances Segment III (System 4)
- Segment I balances Segment III (System 1)
- Segment II balances IV (System 4).

There are no lines connecting Segments 1 to II and IV to III.

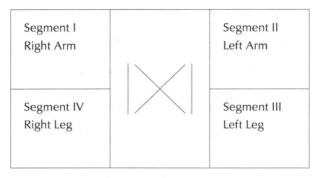

Figure 4.3. Structure B

STRUCTURE C

Figure 4.4 shows that in Structure C, the horizontal lines connect Segments I to II and III to IV. The vertical lines connect Segments I to IV and II to III. Thus:

- Segment I balances Segment II (System 3)
- Segment IV balances Segment III (System 3)
- Segment I balances Segment IV (System 2)
- Segment II balances Segment III (System 4).

The meridians that are selected for treatment must satisfy structure C.

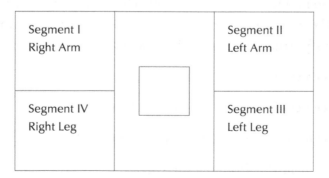

Figure 4.4. Structure C

STRUCTURE D (THE TRUSS STRUCTURE)

Figure 4.5 shows Structure D, which provides the most harmonious and perfect balance not only in engineering terms but also in BM acupuncture. The horizontal lines connect Segments I to II and III to IV. The vertical lines connect Segments I to IV and II to III. The diagonal lines connect Segments I to III and II to IV. Dr Tan's Twelve Magical Points is an excellent example of the Truss Structure, where all the meridians balance one another beautifully:

- Segment I balances Segment II (System 3)
- Segment III balances Segment IV (System 3)
- Segment I balances Segment IV (Systems 2 and 4)
- Segment II balances Segment III (System 2)
- Segment I balances Segment III (System 1)
- Segment II balances Segment IV (System 1).

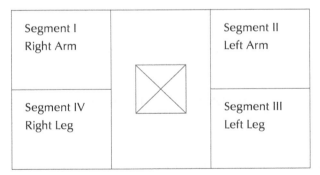

Figure 4.5. Structure D (the Truss Structure)

DYNAMIC BALANCE

The movement in Dynamic Balance reflects the movement in nature, such as the sequential changing of the seasons and day to night. Thus, accordingly, the meridians chosen for treatment must alternate on each limb following the dynamic Yin–Yang–Yin–Yang flow. This notion is based on the Taiji, or Yin–Yang symbol, which is always dynamically balancing itself. In the Taiji, Yin transforms into Yang and Yang into Yin, just as night follows day and day follows night. Two possible patterns are demonstrated in Figures 4.6 and 4.7.

Figure 4.6 follows the Yin–Yang–Yin–Yang meridian flow in a clockwise fashion. It starts with a Yin meridian and ends with a Yang meridian. Figure 4.7 begins with the Yang–Yin–Yang–Yin flow in a clockwise fashion. It starts with a Yang and ends with a Yin meridian.

I Right Arm Yin	II Left Arm Yang
IV Right Leg Yang	III Left Leg Yin

Figure 4.6. Dynamic Balance Clockwise meridian flow: Yin–Yang–Yin–Yang

I Right Arm Yang	II Left Arm Yin
IV Right Leg Yin	III Left Leg Yang

Figure 4.7. Dynamic Balance: Clockwise meridian flow: Yang–Yin–Yang–Yin

THE THREE-STEP ALGORITHM

1. Diagnose the sick meridian(s).

2. Balance the sick meridian(s): Pick from the twelve meridians to create a structure that is based on the Dynamic and Static Balance.

3. Point selection:

    a. Mirror Method

    b. Image Method

    c. Meridian conversion.

Note that in Step 3, I have added meridian conversion for use in the Global Balance Method. So let's take a brief look at the meridian conversion method.

MERIDIAN CONVERSION
What is a hexagram (Ba Gua)?

This method of choosing points for treatment is based on the hexagram (Ba Gua), which is the central balance element of the *I Ching* theory. It is based on the relationship between two hexagrams and their corresponding acupuncture meridians. A hexagram is also called a 'Gua', which means a 'symbol' and 'Ba', which means 'eight'. There are six lines in each hexagram and each line has its own number and name designation. Tables 4.1 and 4.2 show the lines of the hexagram and the primary Yin and Yang meridians respectively. The lines represent the meridians and acupuncture points that are important in meridian conversion.

The aim of this conversion is to switch the sick meridian to the healthy meridian, which results in converting the energies of one meridian into another. Once the conversion has been done, we can select the points for needling, and by so doing we change the condition of the needled meridian, thus bringing it back to a balanced state.

Yin and Yang lines

You need to know these two types of lines: the Yin line, symbolized by two separate horizontal lines ＿ ＿ , and the Yang line, symbolized by one horizontal line ＿＿＿. For example, the LR hexagram has six Yin lines (see Table 4.1) and the GB hexagram has six Yang lines (see Table 4.2). Counting from the bottom line in Table 4.1, LR 1 is a Jing

Well point; LR 2, a Ying Spring point; LR 3, a Shu Stream point; LR 4, Jing River; LR 5, a Luo point; and LR 8, a He Sea point. Likewise, counting from the bottom in Table 4.2, GB 44 is a Jing Well point; GB 43, a Ying Spring point; GB 41, a Shu Stream point; GB 40, a Yuan Source point; GB 38, a Jing River point; and GB 34, a He Sea point.

Table 4.1. Hexagrams and the primary Yin meridians

Lines of hexagram	LR	HT	SP	LU	KI	PC
6 He Sea	8	3	9	5	10	3
5	5 Luo	4 Jing River	5 Jing River	7 Luo	7 Jing River	5 Jing River
4	4 Jing River	5 Luo	4 Luo	8 Jing River	4 Luo	6 Luo
3 Shu Stream	3	7	3	9	3	7
2 Ying Spring	2	8	2	10	2	8
1 Jing Well	1	9	1	11	1	9

Table 4.2. Hexagrams and the primary Yang meridians

Lines of hexagram	GB	SI	ST	LI	UB	TH
6 He Sea	34	8	36	11	40	10
5 Jing River	38	5	41	5	60	6
4 Yuan Source	40	4	42	4	64	4
3 Shu Stream	41	3	43	3	65	3
2 Ying Spring	43	2	44	2	66	2
1 Jing Well	44	1	45	1	67	1

Steps to performing meridian conversion

1. Place the 'sick' meridian (LR) and its associated hexagram next to the healthy hexagram (LI) and its associated hexagram, so that all six lines of each hexagram are next to each other and lined up appropriately, as shown in Table 4.3.

2. Compare the LR hexagram with the LI hexagram. Identify the lines that differ in polarity from the bottom up. Lines 1 and 4 differ from one another. Thus the points to be needled are LR 1 and LR 4, when converting the LR meridian into the LI meridian; and LI 1 and LI 4, when converting the LI meridian into the LR meridian.

Table 4.3. Meridian conversion: comparing the
LR hexagram with the LI hexagram

LR 8	— —	LI 11	— —
LR 5	— —	LI 5	— —
LR 4	— —	LI 4	———
LR 3	— —	LI 3	— —
LR 2	— —	LI 2	— —
LR 1	— —	LI 1	———

EXAMPLES OF MERIDIAN CONVERSION

We can perform conversion in the Global Balance Method in several patterns, such as Tai Yin–Yang Ming, Shao Yin–Shao Yang, Jue Yin–Shao Yang or Jue Yin–Yang Ming. When we do meridian conversion in Global Balance, we convert the hand meridian into the foot meridian and vice versa; we convert the Yang meridian to the Yin meridian and vice versa, thus maintaining the hand ↔ foot, foot ↔ hand, Yin ↔ Yang, Yang ↔ Yin. I've picked a couple of common conditions that are associated with chronic pelvic pain to demonstrate how to perform meridian conversion.

Meridian conversion example 1: Tai Yin–Yang Ming pattern

Many of my patients with chronic pelvic pain also complained of gastrointestinal problems such as IBS, digestive issues (abdominal bloating, nausea, constipation alternating with loose stools), painful bladder, asthma and general fatigue. These symptoms are indicative of an imbalance in the LU, LI, ST and SP meridians, and point to a Tai Yin–Yang Ming pattern. Here are the steps to perform meridian conversion in order to arrive at the points for needling.

Step 1: Ensure that one of the two conditions for Global Balance is satisfied, in this instance Static Balance (Structure A) (see Figure 4.8).

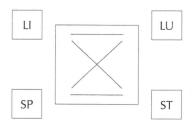

Figure 4.8. Structure A, Static Balance

Steps 2 and 3: To compare the two hexagrams, place them next to each, other as demonstrated earlier (see Figures 4.9–4.11).

Note: Conversion is from hand → foot, foot → hand and Yin → Yang, Yang → Yin.

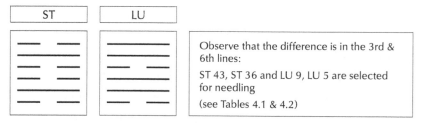

Figure 4.9. Points selected for treatment

The treatment points we have are shown in Figures 4.10 and 4.11, as follows:

THE GLOBAL BALANCE METHOD

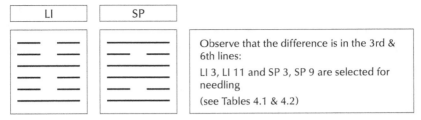

Figure 4.10. Points selected for treatment

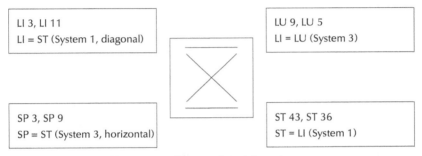

Figure 4.11. Points selected for treatment

EXPLANATION

The meridians involved in the Tai Yin–Yang Ming pattern are LU, SP and LI, ST. Comparing the ST and LU meridians from the bottom line up, note the difference in the 3rd and 6th lines (see Tables 4.1 and 4.2). The points for treatment are LI 3 and LI 11, SP 3 and SP 9. We have now selected eight points for needling. These are the Shu Stream points (LU 9, SP 3 and ST 43, LI 3) and He Sea points (SP 9, LU 5 and ST 36, LI 11).

ADAPTING TAI YIN–YANG MING FOR CHRONIC PELVIC PAIN

I often look for Ashi points around the identified acupuncture points to treat the patient's most serious symptoms. For example, if the chronic pelvic pain is the most bothersome symptom, I adjust the points following the Image Method (Step 3, the lower leg images the lower abdomen). For example, if the pain is in the lower abdomen, with the SP and ST being the sick meridians, I palpate these meridians on the legs where the Ashi points may be around SP 9 and SP 6 and

ST 40 and ST 36 (System 6, using the same meridian to treat itself). I also look for Ashi points on the lower arms along the LU and LI meridians. The Tai Yin–Yang Ming pattern can also be rotated from treatment session to treatment session (see Figure 4.12).

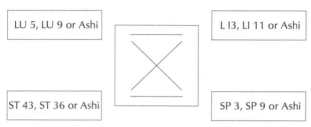

Note that the points needled are the Ashi points and not the exact location as per acupuncture textbooks.

Figure 4.12. Adapting the selected Tai Yin–Yang Ming treatment points for chronic pelvic pain

Meridian conversion example 2: Shao Yang–Tai Yin pattern

Another set of symptoms that I see often in my clinic are irregular bleeding, bloating associated with food and menstruation, breast tenderness, mood swings, water retention, forgetfulness and sleep disorders. These symptoms show that the SP, HT, LR and GB are out of balance. This is basically a Shao Yang–Tai Yin problem with heart disturbance. It could be said in biomedicine that these symptoms point to hormonal imbalance, which is one of the most common problems in women with endometriosis-associated chronic pelvic pain.

Step 1: Ensure that one of the two conditions for Global Balance is satisfied, in this instance Static Balance (Structure B) (see Figure 4.13).

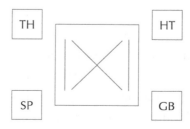

Figure 4.13. Structure B, Static Balance

THE GLOBAL BALANCE METHOD

We satisfy the Static Balance condition where HT balances GB (and vice versa), HT balances SP (and vice versa), and GB balances TH (and vice versa). Note that TH does not balance HT and SP does not balance GB.

Step 2: To compare the two hexagrams, place them next to each other (see Figures 4.14–4.16).

Note: Conversion is from hand → foot, foot → hand and Yin → Yang, Yang → Yin.

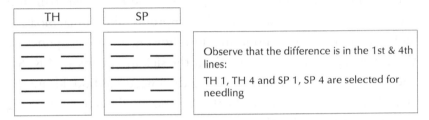

Figure 4.14. Points selected for treatment

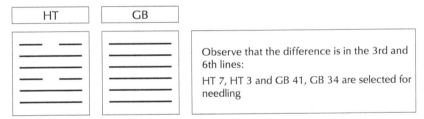

Figure 4.15. Points selected for treatment

Thus, the treatment is as follows:

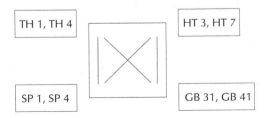

Figure 4.16. The final treatment points

DR TAN'S EIGHT AND TWELVE MAGICAL POINTS

Dr Tan called these two sets of strategies the Eight and Twelve Magical Points, which showcase the Truss Structure (D) of perfect and harmonious balance. The conversion for the Eight Magical Points has already been undertaken.

Dr Tan's Eight Magical Points treatment

The Eight Magical Points (see Figure 4.17) is indicated for gynaecological problems such as infertility, low libido and hormonal imbalance. Again, I adapt this treatment pattern to address pelvic pain and symptoms such as nausea or IBS-like symptoms (abdominal bloating and pain) and hormonal imbalance by following the BM acupuncture three-step algorithm. For example, if the sick meridians are LR, ST and SP (right) lower abdomen, using the Image Method, locate the area, then palpate for and needle the Ashi points along the healthy leg meridians (left) of GB, ST.

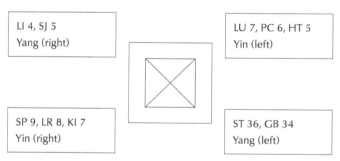

Figure 4.17. Dr Tan's Eight Magical Points

Dr Tan's Twelve Magical Points

This strategy combines the Five Shu points, Yin–Yang Dynamic Balance and Image Method (see Chapter 3). The BM acupuncture three-step algorithm is used when creating a treatment strategy for the Twelve Magical Points:

1. Identify the sick meridian(s) based on the patient's complaints.

2. Identify the healthy meridian(s).

3. Identify the Ashi points on the healthy meridians for treatment using the Image Method to create a group of points in this format: Yin–Yang–Yin–Yang or Yin–Yang–Yin to reflect the Yin–Yang Dynamic Balance.

THE FIVE SHU POINTS

Table 4.4 shows the Five Yin and Yang Shu points of the twelve primary meridians: the Jing Well, Ying Spring, Shu Stream, Jing River and He Sea.

Jing Well points

The Jing Well points are located at the fingers, LU 11, PC 9, HT 9 (Yin) and LI 1, TH 1, SI 1 (Yang). The Jing Well points that are located at the toes are SP 1, LR 1, KI 1 (Yin) and ST 45, GB 44, UB 67 (Yang).

Ying Spring points

The Ying Spring points, which are located in the palm, are LU 10, PC 8, HT 8 (Yin) and LI 2, TH 2, SI 2 (Yang). The Ying Spring points that are located in the medial to the arch of the feet and the top areas are SP 2, LR 2, KI 2 (Yin) and ST 44, GB 43, UB 66 (Yang).

Table 4.4. The Five Yin and Yang Shu points of the upper and lower limbs

Upper and lower limbs	Jing Well	Ying Spring	Shu Stream	Jing River	He Sea
Yin					
LU	LU 11	LU 10	LU 9	LU 8	LU 5
PC	PC 9	PC 8	PC 7	PC 5	PC 3
HT	HT 9	HT 8	HT 7	HT 4	HT 3
SP	SP 1	SP 2	SP 3	SP 5	SP 9
LR	LR 1	LR 2	LR 3	LR 4	LR 8
KI	KI 1	KI 2	KI 3	KI 7	KI 10

Upper and lower limbs	Jing Well	Ying Spring	Shu Stream	Jing River	He Sea
Yang					
LI	LI 1	LI 2	LI 3	LI 5	LI 11
TH	TH 1	TH 2	TH 3	TH 6	TH 10
SI	SI 1	SI 2	SI 3	SI 5	SI 8
ST	ST 45	ST 44	ST 43	ST 41	ST 36
GB	GB 44	GB 43	GB 41	GB 38	GB 34
UB	UB 67	UB 66	UB 65	UB 60	UB 40

Source: Deadman, Al-Khafaji and Baker (2001)

Shu Stream points

The Shu Stream points that are located near the wrists are LU 9, PC 7, HT 7 (Yin) and LI 3, TH 3, SI 3 (Yang). The Shu Stream points located near the ankles are SP 3, LR 3, KI 3 (Yin) and ST 43, GB 41, UB 65 (Yang).

Jing River points

The Jing River points that are located just above and proximal to the wrists are LU 8, PC 5, HT 4 (Yin) and LI 5, TH 6, SI 5 (Yang). The Jing River points that are located near the ankles are SP 5, LR 4, KI 7 (Yin) and ST 41, GB 38, UB 60 (Yang).

He Sea points

The He Sea points that are located around the elbows are LU 5, PC 3, HT 3 (Yin) and LI 11, TH 10, SI 8 (Yang). The He Sea points that are located around the knees are SP 9, LR 8, KI 10 (Yin) and ST 36, GB 34, UB 40 (Yang).

Each group consists of three Shu points with Yin and Yang characteristics, making a total of twelve. Dr Tan called these points the Twelve Magical Points.

Grouping the Five Shu points

We can create four groups from the Five Shu points:

Group 1: Choose a combination of points from the Jing Well and/or Ying Spring points: three from the Jing Well and/or Ying Spring points from the hand Yin and hand Yang and foot Yin and foot Yang meridians: LU 11, PC 9, HT 9 (hand Yin Jing Well), LI 2, TH 2, SI 2 (hand Yang Ying Spring) or ST 45, GB 44, UB 67 (foot Yang Jing Well) and SP 1, LR 1, KI 1 (foot Yin Jing Well). Based on the Image and Reverse Image Method, these points treat the testicles, external genitalia in women, the anus and the top of the head.

Group 2: Choose a combination of points from the Ying Spring and/or Shu Stream points: three hand Yin and hand Yang and three foot Yin and Yang points: LU 9, PC 7, HT 7 (hand Yin), SP 3, LR 3, KI 3 (foot Yin), LI 2, TH 2, SI 2 (hand Yang) and ST 44, GB 43, UB 66 (foot Yang). Based on the Image and Reverse Image Method, these points treat the genitals, coccyx, sacrum and the head, as well as the base of the skull respectively.

Group 3: Choose a combination of points from the Shu Stream and/or Jing River points: LU 9, PC 7, HT 7 (hand Yin), SP 3, LR 3, KI 3 (foot Yin), LI 3, TH 3, SI 3 (hand Yang) and ST 43, GB 41, UB 65 (foot Yang). Based on the Image and Reverse Image Method, these points treat the lower abdomen, lower back and upper abdomen, rib cage and upper-mid back respectively.

Group 4: Choose a combination of points from the Jing River and/or He Sea points: LU 8, PC 5, HT 4 (hand Yin), SP 5, LR 4, KI 7 (leg Yin), LI 5, TH 6, SI 5 (hand Yang) and ST 36, GB 34, UB 40 (foot Yang). Based on the Image and Reverse Image Method, these points treat the level of the umbilicus, lumbar 2 and waist.

Point selection: Image Method

This is Step 2 of the Twelve Magical Points treatment strategy. Although I described the Image and Reverse Image Methods of point selection in Chapter 3, for convenience I have presented them again here, in Table 4.5.

Table 4.5. The Image Method

To be needled	Image Method (affected area)	Reverse Image Method (affected area)
Finger/Toe	Testicles, external genitalia (women), anus	Top of head
Hand/Foot	Genitals, coccyx, sacrum	Head, base of skull
Wrist/Ankle	Bladder, lumbosacral area	Neck, neck joint
Forearm/Lower leg	Lower abdomen, lower back	Upper abdomen, rib cage, mid-upper back
Elbow/Knee	Umbilicus level, lumbar 2, waist	Umbilicus level, lumbar 2, waist
Upper arm/Upper leg	Upper abdomen, rib cage, chest, mid-upper back	Lower abdomen, lower back
Shoulder/Hip joint	Neck, jaw, base of skull	Sacrum, genitals, coccyx
Top of shoulder/Top of hip	Top of head	Testicles, external genitalia (women), anus

Yin–Yang Dynamic Balance of the twelve meridians

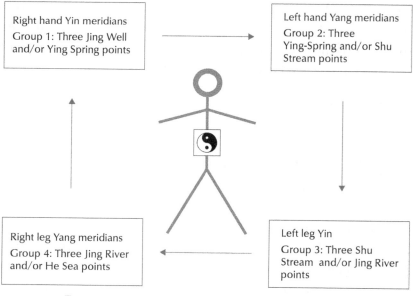

Figure 4.18. Yin–Yang Dynamic Balance, four groups of points with alternating Yin–Yang–Yin–Yang

Figure 4.18 shows a Yin–Yang Dynamic Balance where a group of three Yin meridians is followed by a group of Yang, then Yin and Yang meridians: Yin → Yang → Yin → Yang. Alternatively one can start with a Yang → Yin → Yang → Yin. This is Step 3 of the Twelve Magical Points treatment strategy.

Figure 4.19 shows:

Group 1, Segment 1, right arm:

- LU 11, PC 9, HT 9 (all Jing Well points) *or*

- LU 10, HT 8, PC 8 (all Ying Spring points) *or*

- LU 10, HT 9, PC 8 (a mix of Jing Well and Ying Spring points).

Using the Image Method, these points treat the testicles, external genitalia in women, the anus and the top of the head.

Group 2, Segment 2, left arm:

- LI 2, SI 2, TH 2 (all Ying Spring points) *or*

- LI 3, SI 3, TH 3 (all Shu Stream points) *or*

- LI 3, SI 2, TH 2 (a mix of Shu Stream and Ying Spring points).

Using the Image Method, these points treat the genitals, coccyx, sacrum and the head and base of the skull.

Group 3, Segment 3, left leg:

- KI 3, LR 3, SP 3 (all Shu Stream points) *or*

- KI 7, LR 4, SP 5 (all Jing River points) *or*

- KI 3, LR 4, SP 3 (a mix of Shu Stream and Jing River points).

Using the Image Method, these points treat the lower abdomen, lower back, upper abdomen, rib cage and upper-mid back.

Group 4, Segment 4, right leg:

- UB 60, ST 41, GB 38 (all Jing River points) *or*
- UB 40, ST 36, GB 34 (all Shu Stream points) *or*
- UB 60, ST 36, GB 38 (a mix of Shu Stream and Jing River points).

Using the Image Method, these treat the level of the umbilicus, lumbar 2 and waist.

Using the same four groups of points you can create *eight clockwise* patterns. Each of the eight patterns can be flipped to the opposite side of the body (*anti-clockwise patterns*), to make up 16 different combinations.

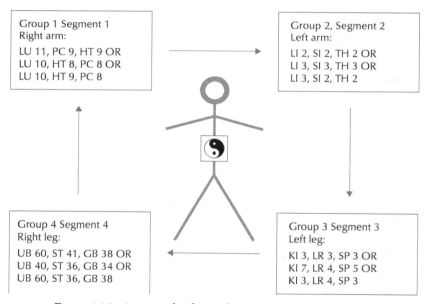

Figure 4.19. An example of a Twelve Magical Points treatment

How to adapt the Twelve Magical Points for chronic pelvic pain

CASE STUDY 1

This patient has endometriosis-associated pelvic pain (see Figure 4.20). Her complaints, in order of seriousness, are as follows: severe

THE GLOBAL BALANCE METHOD

endometriosis-associated left pelvic pain, with bloating and nausea (9/10, 10 being most painful), right neck pain (5/10) and a vague left low back pain, fatigue, depression, anxiety and insomnia.

Treating chronic pelvic pain (left), bloating and nausea
Follow the three-steps algorithm:

1. Identify the sick meridians: SP, LR, KI, ST (left).

2. Identify the healthy meridians: ST, GB, UB (right).

3. Identify the Ashi points on the healthy meridians for treatment using the Image Method: ST 36, GB 34, UB 40 (right leg, Group 4).

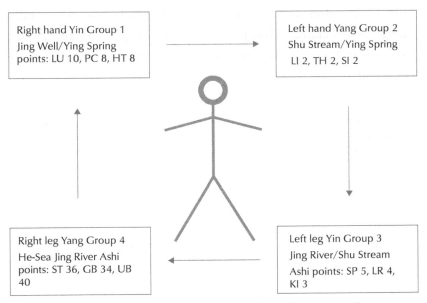

Figure 4.20. Yin–Yang Dynamic Balance, four groups of points with alternating Yin–Yang–Yin–Yang

Treating right neck pain

1. Identify the sick meridians: GB, SI, UB.

2. Identify the healthy meridians to balance the sick meridians: LR, SP, KI.

3. Select Ashi points using the Reverse Image Method: Palpate for and needle the Ashi points (ankle reverse images neck and neck joint): SP 5, LR 4, KI 3 (left leg, Group 3).

In accordance with Dr Tan's Twelve Magical Points treatment, I completed the missing Groups 1 and 2. Once all the needles were inserted, the patient reported a sense of peace and calmness, accompanied by a slowing of the breath. Her pelvic pain level and bloating were reduced significantly, as was her left low back pain.

CASE STUDY 2

In order of seriousness, this patient complains of: right-sided endometriosis-associated pelvic pain 9/10 (10 being most painful) and right-sided knee pain (6/10), poor digestion and vertex headache (see Figure 4.21).

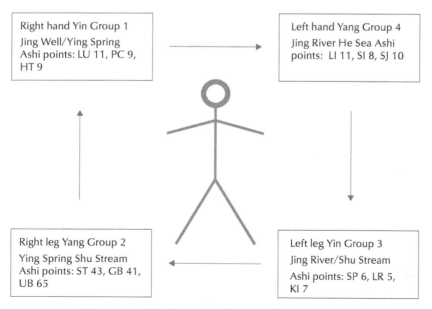

Figure 4.21. Twelve Magical Points of four groups of points with alternating Yin–Yang–Yin–Yang

Treating chronic pelvic pain (right)

1. Identify the sick meridians: ST, SP, GB, KI (right).

2. Identify the healthy meridians to balance the sick meridians: SP, LR.

3. Identify the Ashi points on the healthy meridians using the Image Method: Ashi points around SP 6 and LR 5 (KI 7 is added for Global Balance) (left leg, Group 3).

Treating right knee pain

1. Identify the sick meridians: ST, GB, UB (right).

2. Identify the healthy meridians to balance the sick meridians: LI, TH, SI.

3. Select treatment points using the Mirror Method: palpate for and needle the Ashi points around LI 11, SI 8 and TH 10.

Following Dr Tan's Twelve Magical Point strategy, I then added the missing Groups 1 and 2.

CONCLUDING THOUGHTS

Thus far I have presented the Global Balance Method and Dr Tan's Twelve Magical Points. In my clinical practice, I use the Twelve Magical Points regularly, and many of my patients find this strategy helpful in relieving their symptoms. In treating patients with complex presentations, and when indicated, I integrate the techniques of Alchemical Healing (Chapter 7) and Five Elements acupuncture (Chapter 6), which are really useful.

I would like to conclude this chapter by leaving a few useful clinical pearls for my readers.

CLINICAL PEARLS

- It is crucial to palpate for and treat the Ashi points. In BM acupuncture, the exact textbook point location is not so important.

- To obtain the best result, it is important to achieve De Qi (a heavy, distending sensation felt by the patient), because this is crucial to the success of the treatment.

- It is also important to stimulate the needles.

- I leave the needles in for at least 30 minutes, although Dr Tan suggested leaving them for about 45–60 minutes for the best result.

— CHAPTER 5 —

TRIGGER POINTS

INTRODUCTION

For some women, their chronic pelvic pain could be due to or aggravated by trigger points. Most of the patients I treat in my pelvic pain clinic usually have a known cause such as endometriosis, although they often develop trigger points that can confuse the symptom presentation. These trigger points may be a missing piece of the puzzle, in which case deactivating them may help to relieve the pain. It is thus useful to learn more about trigger points and what you can do to reduce the pain they produce.

WHAT ARE TRIGGER POINTS?

Trigger points are gummy, contracted, exquisitely tender bands of muscle tissue (Davies and Davies 2013, p.10). They are not only tender to palpate, but they also have a specific referral pain pattern to other parts of the body. Referred pain is a characteristic of a trigger point upon palpation that differentiates it from a tender point (an Ashi point), which is painful only at the area of palpation. Another characteristic of a trigger point is a local twitch response that is elicited when palpating perpendicularly to the muscle fibres in a snapping or plucking manner, using the thumb and index finger. A local twitch response is a transient visible or palpable contraction of the muscle and skin.

Trigger points can be active or latent. Active trigger points are pathological, and are usually painful regardless of whether they are in an active or passive state as the muscle fibres are in a chronically contracted condition. Take, for example, trigger points in the piriformis muscle. Weight bearing on the affected leg (active state) could cause the piriformis muscle to further tighten, creating a sensation of pain. Pain is also felt during active stretching, as in a figure-of-four stretch (a stretch that can be done lying down with the left ankle positioned just above a bent right knee, and with both hands gently pulling or holding the right lower leg, until the stretch is felt). Likewise, pain can be present during a passive state such as when lying down at rest. Latent trigger points do not usually produce pain but will do so if the patient is physically and/or emotionally stressed (Davies and Davies 2013).

Trigger points are also known as myofascial trigger points – 'myo' refers to the muscle and 'fascia' to the connective tissue. Those who include meat in their diet, and have experience handling an uncooked piece of chicken, will have noticed that between the skin and the meat (muscle) is a transparent, slippery and smooth film – this is the fascia. It encloses and binds together muscles, blood vessels, lymphatic vessels and nerves. It is the nerve supply that makes the fascia tender. Imagine a three-dimensional elasticated wrap – the fascia envelops all our internal organs from head to toe, giving stability and allowing them to glide smoothly over each other. This is a description of a healthy fascia. In contrast, an unhealthy fascia is thick and inflexible or dries up around the muscles, limiting mobility and causing painful knots to develop. Muscles that have trigger points can tighten and shrink and are usually stiff and weak and have a limited range of motion. Besides chronic pelvic pain, trigger points can cause or aggravate wide-ranging problems such as headache, tinnitus and changes in balance and coordination (Davies and Davies 2013, Chapter 4). Therefore, it is an excellent idea to know your trigger points and to keep your muscles and fascia healthy by eating a healthy and balanced diet as well as engaging in physical activities such as Yoga (discussed in Chapters 8 and 9).

Some common predisposing factors to developing trigger points are lack of or overexercise and repetitive exercise, occupational activities that require repetitive actions, chronic sleep disturbances as well as scars due to surgery or inflammation (Grosman-Rimon *et al.* 2016).

ARE TRIGGER POINTS ASHI POINTS?

Acupuncturists will recognize that trigger points are very similar to Ashi points, but they are not the same. The needling technique for Ashi points is totally different from the technique involved in deactivating a trigger point. Ashi points are described as tight and tender, but do not cause referred pain, unlike trigger points. Among acupuncturists, Ashi points are commonly understood as the patient's response to the painful area being palpated – 'a' as in the shout from the patient when the tender area is being palpated and 'shi' (meaning 'yes' in spoken Chinese) as confirmation of the tender spot. Jiang and Zhao (2016), however, point out that 'Ashi' refers to the popular method of treatment used by ordinary folks in China over 2000 years ago, implying that it is so easy to treat that the layperson can get rid of the pain by treating the Ashi points themselves. And it is indeed possible to do this by such methods as Yamuna body rolling, Yin Yoga, intentional breathing or other self-care techniques outlined in this book (see Chapter 9). This is especially useful for patients who are needle-sensitive, or where trigger points are difficult to access and thus cannot be safely deactivated using an acupuncture needle.

Trigger points that aggravate or cause chronic pelvic pain

Trigger points in the general population are more common than we think. It is estimated that between 14 and 23 per cent of women with chronic pelvic pain have trigger points (Tu, As-Sanie and Steege 2006). It is commonly believed, but mistakenly so, that chronic pelvic pain is almost always due to a problem with an internal organ. Therefore, it comes as a surprise to many patients that trigger points can be the cause of chronic pelvic pain or part of the problem. For example, trigger points in the pelvic floor muscles, pelvic wall muscles (the piriformis and obturator internus), abdominal muscles, adductor magnus muscle and iliopsoas muscle are the most common ones to cause or aggravate chronic pelvic pain in women (Travell and Simons 1993).

As it is beyond the scope of this chapter to cover all the muscles and trigger points of the body, this chapter will focus on these muscles in particular. I can, however, further recommend two essential books that I find very helpful. The most useful source on muscles and bones is Andrew Biel's *Trail Guide to the Body: A Hands-On Guide to Locating Muscles, Bones, and More* (3rd edn, Handspring Publishing, 2005). A book on trigger points by Clair Davies and Amber Davies, *The Trigger Point Therapy Workbook: Your Self-Treatment Guide for Pain Relief* (3rd edn, New Harbinger, 2004), is invaluable and easy to follow. Further, there are useful trigger point charts that are more affordable or available for download from some websites, although there aren't many.[10]

A CLASSICAL CHINESE ACUPUNCTURE APPROACH TO DEACTIVATING TRIGGER POINTS

I cannot really talk about trigger points without acknowledging the work of Dr Janet Travell and Dr David Simons as well as Dr Mark Seem, licensed acupuncturist and founder of the Tri-State College of Acupuncture, New York City. Travell and Simons published a two-volume manual, *Myofascial Pain and Dysfunction: The Trigger Point Manual* (Simons, Travell and Simons 1999; Travell and Simons 1993), in which they explored, in great detail, trigger points, referred pain and treatment methods. In one of the treatment methods, Dr Travell typically employed a thick 3–5 inch long syringe to inject lidocaine into the trigger point. Following on from Dr Travell's work, Dr Seem developed an excellent technique to release trigger points that he called a classical Chinese acupuncture needling approach using a thin and short acupuncture needle, such as a Japanese Seirin J-Type needle (34–36 gauge x 40mm/1.58 inches). This form of trigger point release is also known as dry needling.

Dr Seem taught us to insert the acupuncture needle slowly and superficially over but not into the trigger point, until the needle meets with some resistance. This is followed by several gentle pecks into the resistance with the needle, whereupon the muscle usually twitches and grabs the needle. This process of deactivating a trigger point is facilitated by compressing the soft tissue with the practitioner's non-needling hand, loosening up occasionally to encourage the deep muscle to react with a twitch. This is usually felt as a muscle contraction for a few seconds by the patient. The practitioner can also see the twitch and feel it with the non-needling hand. The twitching encourages the stretching of the tight contracted muscle and the releasing of the trigger point. This twitching response is believed to be the mechanism by which trigger points are deactivated. This method of using a classical Chinese acupuncture needling approach is one that I learned from Dr Seem and his team while I was a student at the Tri-State College of Acupuncture. It is a safe way to release a trigger point as you can see that the acupuncture needle is relatively short and the needling depth is relatively shallow (Seem 1993).

Over the years, in addition to learning the anatomy of the body, I have found that careful preparation of my patients and myself is paramount to the success of deactivating trigger points successfully and safely. In creating trust, this further helps with establishing and maintaining a positive relationship, which has been shown to be therapeutic.

PREPARING THE PATIENT FOR PALPATION AND TRIGGER POINT RELEASE

- Baseline pain level: If you have not done so already, this is a good time to ask the patient to rate their pain level using the visual analogue scale (VAS), as shown in Figure 5.1. This is a validated (shown to be accurate), subjective measure for pain with a continuous scale starting from '0 (no pain) to 10 (worst pain)' (Bond and Pilowsky 1966). Patients are instructed to mark a number on the line that corresponds to their current pain level, which forms the pre-treatment baseline. By comparing this pain baseline with the post-treatment pain level, this gives us an idea of the effectiveness of the trigger point release treatment.

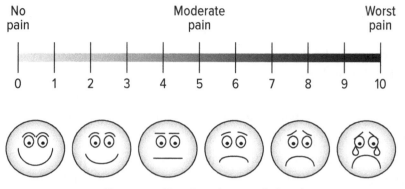

Figure 5.1. Visual analogue scale (VAS)

- Visual images: I find it helpful for the patient to be shown the appropriate trigger point referral pain pattern(s) from a trigger point flip chart. Visual images give the patient a useful practical guide to understanding their pain pattern. I find that most of the time patients can quickly identify their trigger point's pain pattern when shown the appropriate ones. Further, they also help to refresh your memory of trigger point referral patterns.

- Breathwork: It is equally important to encourage the patient to focus on their breath-in and breath-out to help them relax before you start the palpation and treatment.

- Useful information: The patient should be informed that you are looking for a tender, contracted and knotty, tight area in a band of muscle and that the pain can be reproduced when you press on it. This is a good thing because it means that you have found the trigger point.

- Positive reinforcement: Inform the patient that when the trigger point is being treated, they may feel an involuntary twitch in the muscle. This twitch response is a positive sign as it shows that the painful contracted muscle has been deactivated. As a result, the muscle fibres will soften, leading to a reduction in pain. The treated area will feel achy, which is often described as a 'post-exercise' sensation, and will continue to relax over the following 24 hours or so.

Post treatment

- Needle retention: After the twitching, and once the muscles have softened, remove the needle. I usually wait 5–10 minutes before I remove the needle, especially if the area I am working on is the lower abdomen as the muscle can begin to tighten again and can cause pain if the needle is left in place for too long. This is why it is very important to continue to remind the patient to focus on the breath-in and breath-out, to discourage the muscles from tightening.

- Epsom salt bath and fluid intake: Advise the patient to drink plenty of fluids after the treatment and to take a bath with Epsom salt, which will further help with muscle relaxation.

- Questions: Give the patient plenty of opportunity to ask questions.

PREPARATION FOR THE HEALTHCARE PROFESSIONAL

Steps 1–3 below are fundamental. Grounding yourself and having a comfortable posture provides a link between you and the patient as well as what you are trying to achieve. If you are not grounded, sometimes the act of deactivating the trigger point can be a shock to both you and the patient, especially if the twitch response is strong. Palpation depth and knowledge of anatomy are crucial to deactivating a trigger point successfully and safely. Always be aware of what arteries, nerves or veins are near the trigger point(s) that are being treated:

1. Be comfortable: ensure the examining table is the right height for you and that your posture is well supported by standing with feet hip distance apart. If it is more comfortable, you may prefer to sit on a comfortable treatment stool.

2. Centre or ground yourself: focus on your breath-in and breath-out and create an intention.

3. Focus your attention on your intention for successful palpation and deactivation of the trigger point.

4. I find the best way to palpate is to gently strum my thumb or middle and index fingers over the band of tight muscle. Carefully watch the patient's reaction, as the palpation will reproduce the pain and/or a twitch response. This is a good indication that you have found the trigger point. Once you have found the trigger point, do *not* continue to palate the area as it may irritate the tissue further.

5. Some trigger points are buried deep in the muscle, such as those in the adductor magnus or the iliopsoas. If you are new to trigger points and do not feel comfortable deactivating them, it is best left to the physiotherapist who specializes in pelvic pain. In the meantime, offer helpful self-care advice or home remedies to the patient (discussed in Chapters 8 and 9).

CLASSICAL CHINESE ACUPUNCTURE NEEDLING INSTRUCTIONS TO RELEASE TRIGGER POINT(S)

1. Choose an acupuncture needle you are comfortable working with and prefer. I am used to using a Seirin J-Type needle (diameter and length: 0.25/0.22/0.20 x 40mm).

2. Focus your attention and imagine the position of the trigger point that you are going to deactivate, and remember to breathe.

3. Insert the acupuncture needle slowly and carefully into the soft tissue over the trigger point, but *not* into the trigger point, until you come across resistance.

4. Gently compress the soft tissue with your non-needling hand, loosening up occasionally to allow space for the deep muscle to react.

5. Apply a non-rhythmical, gentle pecking movement with the direction changing so as to 'surprise' the trigger point into a twitching response. (Note: This is in contrast to obtaining the De Qi sensation, which needs a rhythmical in and out twirling technique.)

6. If there is more than one trigger point, repeat the steps from palpation to needle insertion. Proceed with care, as some patients may not be able to tolerate the deactivation of too many trigger points. Always check in with the patient and evaluate the patient's condition.

7. Evaluate the patient by asking them to rate their pain level post treatment using the VAS tool (see Figure 5.1).

8. Remind the patient that the involved muscle will continue to relax over the next 24 hours or so.

Contraindications

- The patient does not consent or is not able to do so. In my experience, this group of patients usually cannot tolerate muscle twitching. It is best not to go ahead with the deactivation of trigger point treatment.

- Active infection over the site of the trigger point.

- The trigger point is difficult to access and cannot be safely deactivated.

Precautions

- The patient who is on anticoagulants (blood thinners). I am very careful with patients who are on anticoagulants, especially if they report easy bruising and bleeding. When in doubt, do not deactivate the trigger point(s). I also press the area of needle insertion for a full minute after the needle has been removed, to ensure that there is no bleeding.

- Pregnant patient. It is always good practice to proceed with care and caution, especially if the patient has never had a trigger point deactivated before.

- Sensitive patient. I have come across very sensitive patients who find muscle twitching uncomfortable but who will tolerate the experience, especially if they know that it will help with their pain.

PELVIC FLOOR MUSCLES TRIGGER POINTS

Imagine the pelvic cavity as a room or a bowl that has a bottom and sides. Just like the floor of a room that supports its contents, the pelvic floor muscle group is designed to do the heavy and important work of supporting the pelvic and abdominal contents. The pelvic floor consists of a group of superficial muscles (urogenital diaphragm) and a group of deep muscles (pelvic diaphragm). Trigger points can develop in these muscles and there are many potential causes for their presence.

Women are at risk of developing trigger points in the pelvic floor muscles during pregnancy and childbirth, as well as after pelvic surgery, infection in the reproductive tract, endometriosis and haemorrhoids. Further, traumatic or vigorous sexual activities are potential causes of trigger points in the pelvic floor.

Overexercising the core muscles (pelvis, lower back, hips and stomach muscles), the pelvic floor muscles during Kegel (an exercise to strengthen the pelvic floor muscles to prevent accidentally passing urine or faeces) and Pilates can lead to tight pelvic floor muscles and

TRIGGER POINTS

the development of trigger points. Inattention to someone's posture, such as sitting, slouched, for a long time on the tailbone, and using bad techniques when lifting heavy weights, add to the long list for the development of trigger points (Davies and Davies 2013).

You can see or feel the most superficial urogenital diaphragm in the area between the anus and the vagina (perineum), the muscles surrounding the vagina, clitoris and anus. This superficial pelvic floor muscle group is also responsible for maintaining urinary, bowel and normal sexual function.

The deep floor muscles (pelvic diaphragm) are formed by a group of muscles called the levator ani, which supports the pelvic organs (bladder, vagina and rectum). The levator ani assists the sphincters of the anus and urethra. Figure 5.2 shows the trigger points and referral pattern of the levator ani, sphincter ani and coccygeus muscle.

Referral pattern: Trigger point(s) in the pelvic floor muscles refer pain to the lower torso.

Symptoms: Painful sexual intercourse, stress incontinence, pain in the vulva, vagina, rectum, anus, bladder, urethra, low back pain, pain in the sacrum and tailbone, as well as pain during menstruation. The pain can be initiated by sitting down or lying flat on one's back, and also during bowel movements.

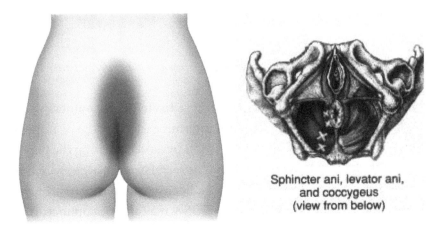

Sphincter ani, levator ani, and coccygeus (view from below)

Figure 5.2. Deep pelvic floor trigger points and pain referral pattern

Inner-side wall pelvic muscles: obturator internus and piriformis

OBTURATOR INTERNUS

The obturator internus (see Figure 5.3) is the deep muscle of the hip joint, and it inserts into the head of the femur, just below the piriformis muscle insertion.

Referral pattern: Trigger point(s) in the obturator internus refer pain to the lower torso.

Symptoms: Pain and a sense of fullness in the rectum, pain in the tailbone and vagina, painful sexual intercourse and menstrual problems.

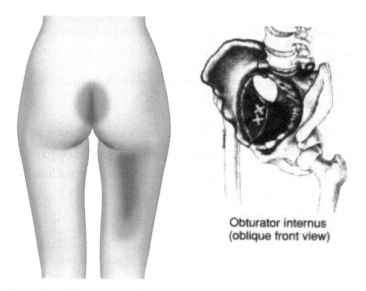

Figure 5.3. Obturator internus trigger points and pain referral pattern

I have never attempted to palpate or deactivate trigger points in pelvic floor muscles and the obturator internus except for the piriformis muscle (pelvic side wall muscles). This is because palpating the pelvic floor muscles involves a vaginal and/or rectal examination, which is beyond the scope of my practice as a licensed acupuncturist in the UK (although countries such as the USA may allow acupuncturists to do this). Nonetheless, it is useful to know that trigger points in the pelvic floor muscles exist. If I suspect that there are trigger points in these muscles, I will always advise my patients to consult a physiotherapist who specializes in trigger points and chronic pelvic pain. In the meantime, it is a good idea to suggest some self-help techniques to the patient (see Chapters 8 and 9).

PIRIFORMIS MUSCLE

The piriformis muscle attaches to the anterior sacrum, and then runs underneath the gluteus maximus and attaches to the bony protrusion of the greater trochanter. The sciatic nerve passes directly below the piriformis (see Figure 5.4).

Referral pattern: Trigger point(s) in the piriformis muscle refer pain to the lower torso.

Symptoms: Painful sexual intercourse, rectum and anal perineum buttock pain, stress incontinence, pain in the side of the thigh and hip pain.

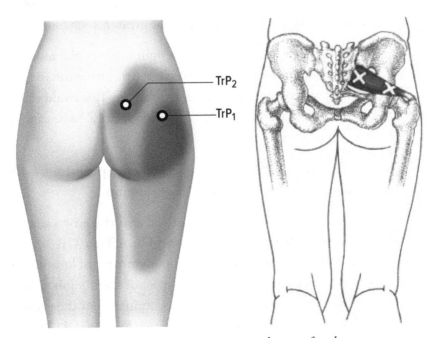

Figure 5.4. Piriformis trigger points and pain referral pattern

Landmarks: Posterior superior iliac spine (PSIS), coccyx (tailbone), sacrum and greater trochanter (hip bone).

1. Position yourself on the same side of the piriformis muscle you are palpating.

2. The patient should preferably be on their stomach, but if this is not possible, position them on their side, with their knees slightly bent.

3. Find these two landmarks: the posterior superior iliac spine (PSIS) and the coccyx (tailbone).

4. Find the third landmark (sacrum). Draw an imaginary line from the PSIS and the coccyx towards the greater trochanter, and where the two lines meet (sacrum) is the attachment of the piriformis (you can now feel the beginning of the piriformis muscle).

5. Find the fourth landmark (greater trochanter). The piriformis is located between the sacrum and the greater trochanter.

6. Now palpate perpendicularly (at a right angle to the muscle) deep into the gluteus maximus muscle, starting from the sacrum and working towards the greater trochanter. This could cause the patient to have a sensation of 'pseudo sciatica', so be careful how you proceed.

7. Palpate with a strumming action along the piriformis for a sensitive, tight band of muscles (trigger points).

8. Acupuncturists will have now noticed that these two trigger points are likely to be found around Huan Tiao/GB 30 and Ju Liao/GB 29. The traditional acupuncture point location of GB 30 is on the posterior-lateral aspect of the hip joint, one-third of the distance between the prominence of the greater trochanter and the sacrococcygeal hiatus (Yao Hu/DU 2). The location of GB 29 is on the 'lateral aspect of the hip joint, at

the midpoint of a line drawn between the anterior superior iliac spine (ASIS) and the prominence of the greater trochanter' (Deadman, Al-Khafaji and Baker 2001, p.446).

Caution

Because the piriformis muscle is near to the sciatic nerve and the pudendal nerve, caution is needed during deactivation of the trigger point using an acupuncture needle. The pudendal nerve originates from sacral nerves 2, 3 and 4, which travel through the piriformis muscle (Weiss 2019). Some patients have an anomalous sciatic nerve that goes through the piriformis. The practitioner can only find this out when deactivating the trigger point, which causes a temporary electrical feeling that shoots down the leg. Thus, go slowly and gently.

ABDOMINAL MUSCLES TRIGGER POINTS

Our abdominal muscles perform many important functions, such as protecting the internal organs, assisting in breathing, coughing, vomiting and opening the bowels, and giving birth and urination. These muscles are arranged vertically and at different angles.

The abdominal muscles that are arranged vertically are the rectus abdominis (commonly called the 'six pack' or 'abs'), which forms the central muscles that stretch from the lower ribs to the pubic bone; the abdominal oblique muscles (on the sides of the abdomen), which originate from the lower ribs and the iliac crest and continue on to the abdominal aponeurosis (the fascia of the rectus abdominis); the inguinal ligament, which connects the front of the pelvis to the pubic bone; and the thoracolumbar fascia (covering the spinal muscles). The abdominal oblique muscles consist of the external oblique, internal oblique and the transverse abdominis.

Trigger points in the abdominal muscles can be caused by stress, fatigue, inflammation and overexertion of the abdominal muscles (e.g., too many abdominal crunches), as well as scar tissue from abdominal surgery.

Upper rectus abdominis trigger points

Referral pattern: The waist area, mid-back and stomach area.

Symptoms: Heart burn, acid reflux, indigestion, nausea and abdominal bloating, which are commonly mistaken as problems in the gastrointestinal tract.

Lower rectus abdominis trigger points

Referral pattern: Low back and sacroiliac joints, which link the iliac bone (pelvis) to the sacrum (lowest part of the spine, just above the tailbone) (see Figure 5.5).

Symptoms: Period pain, pain in the pelvic floor, vagina, ovaries, uterus, anus and rectum, low back pain, spasm and pain in the urinary bladder, and urinary difficulties and frequency. These symptoms can be mistaken for problems in the bladder or reproductive system and the pelvic floor muscles.

Palpating the rectus abdominis muscles and its trigger points

1. Position your patient on their back and yourself on the side of the muscle you are going to palpate.

2. Make sure the patient has emptied their bladder before palpation.

3. Palpate with your fingers and palm in a flat position along the lateral border of the rectus abdominis muscle, starting from the lower abdomen and working to the top.

4. When you find a taut band, stay there for a few more minutes as this might reproduce the patient's pain (e.g., low back pain), and it confirms the presence of a trigger point.

5. Stay on the trigger point for little longer and apply a little more pressure (always get the patient's feedback) as you remind your

patient to take a slow breath-in and breath-out. By doing this, sometimes the trigger point can be released or ameliorated.

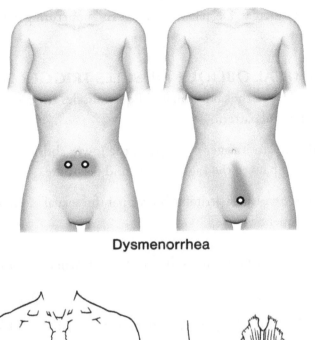

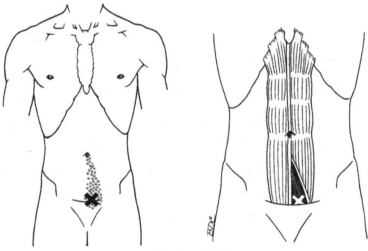

Figure 5.5. Lower rectus abdominis trigger points and pain referral pattern

Caution

When needling this area, remember that there are important organs that are underneath the rectus abdominis muscle, such as the stomach, spleen and pancreas. Deep insertion may risk puncturing these organs.

ABDOMINAL OBLIQUE MUSCLES TRIGGER POINTS

Figure 5.6 shows the abdominal oblique muscles trigger points and the pain referral pattern.

Referral pattern: Trigger point(s) in the lower abdominal oblique muscles refer pain to the vagina, groin and pelvic area.

Symptoms: Diarrhoea, irritable bowel, painful sexual intercourse and urinary frequency.

Palpating the oblique muscles and lower trigger points

1. Position your patient on their back.

2. Make sure the patient has emptied their bladder before palpation.

3. Position yourself on either the right or left side of the patient.

4. Trigger points in the lateral oblique muscles are usually found around Wu Shu/GB 27 and Wei Dao/GB 28.

5. Locate GB 27. Find the anterior superior iliac spine (ASIS). GB 27 is in the depression, just anterior to the ASIS, about 3 cun below the umbilicus. Look for a tight and tender spot around this area.

6. Locate GB 28, which is 0.5 cun anterior and inferior to GB 27. Again, palpate around this area for a tight and tender area.

7. Also look for tightness and tenderness around Dai Mai/GB 26,

which is anterior and inferior to the free end of the 11th rib, level with the umbilicus.

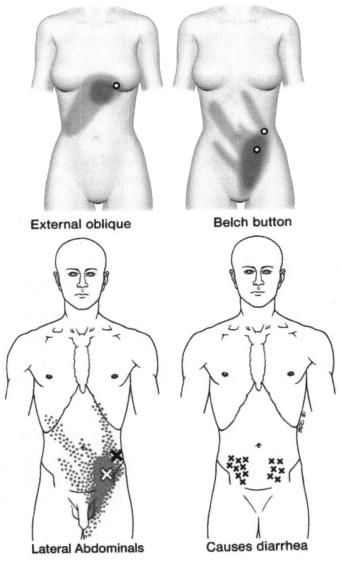

Figure 5.6. Abdominal oblique muscles trigger points and pain referral pattern

ADDUCTOR MAGNUS MUSCLES TRIGGER POINTS

The adductor magnus (see Figure 5.7) is the largest muscle in the adductor group that fans out from under the pubic bone to attach at several points along the femur. It is situated deep in the inner thigh area. The adductor magnus attaches to the pelvis and several points along the femur, and is located in the inner thigh between the hamstring muscle group and the quadriceps muscle group in the front.

Overdoing activities such as climbing stairs, mountains, riding a horse, overstretching while exercising and skiing (making quick turns) can create trigger points in the adductor magnus muscles, as can long bicycle or car trips and sitting with legs crossed for a long time. Patients with trigger points in these muscles describe the pain as sharp and sudden.

Referral pattern: The groin or inner thigh area.

Symptoms: Pain in the hip, inside the pelvis, vagina and rectum, severe menstrual cramping, and pain during and/or after sexual intercourse.

Palpating the adductor magnus muscle and its trigger point

Landmarks: Femur, sacrum, pelvis, gluteal fold.

1. Position the patient on one side with their top leg bent towards the waist and the other one straight (to be palpated).

2. Position yourself behind the patient.

3. The first trigger point is located along the midline of the inner thigh, about halfway between the inner thigh and inner knee. The second trigger point is a couple of inches below the gluteal fold. It is a good idea, however, to palpate along the midline for other possible trigger point(s).

4. This midline is roughly where the Kidney meridian or inner Yin line is.

5. You can massage the trigger point(s) with your elbow or thumbs

and apply gentle pressure on the trigger point if needling is not appropriate.

Caution
Trigger points in the adductor magnus are difficult to access because the muscle is situated deep in the inner thigh. Care must be taken when needling perpendicularly from the medial aspect of the thigh as the sciatic nerve passes close to the adductor magnus (Travell and Simons 1993, p.312). However, it is unlikely to be a problem if you are using the classical Chinese acupuncture needling.

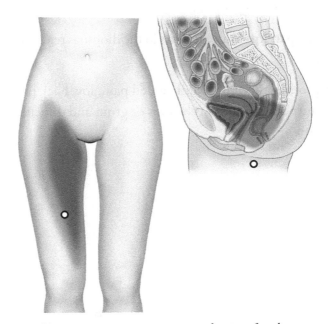

Figure 5.7. Adductor magnus trigger points and pain referral pattern

ILIOPSOAS MUSCLE TRIGGER POINTS
The psoas and iliacus are called the iliopsoas (see Figure 5.8). It is one of the core muscles that is hidden deep behind the abdominal muscles and intestines. The iliacus is the first part of the iliopsoas, which is attached to the iliac bone, and can be found underneath the iliac crest.

The psoas muscle starts at thoracic spine 12 (T12) and attaches itself to lumbar spine L1, L2, L3, L4 and L5. The psoas continues down to the pelvis to join the iliacus in the groin to become the iliopsoas, and then attaches itself inside the lesser trochanter. If you are not sure what this muscle looks like, when you are next in a supermarket, look for a tenderloin or filet mignon; you are looking at the iliopsoas (of a cow or pig).

Because the iliopsoas is a core muscle, any strenuous exercises such as abdominal crunches, sit-ups, leg-ups, gruelling running or walking that overworks the psoas can cause trigger points and/or further aggravate the trigger points that are already present.

Referral pattern: Trigger points in the iliopsoas refer pain to the lower body.

Symptoms: Abdominal and genital pain, low back pain and pain in the buttocks, stiffness in the hips or groin and difficulty standing up straight.

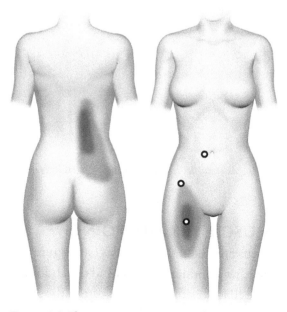

Figure 5.8. Iliopsoas trigger points and pain referral pattern

Palpating the iliopsoas muscle and its trigger point(s)

Landmarks: Anterior superior iliac spine (ASIS), inguinal ligament that runs down the pubic bone, inside the leg (lesser trochanter).

1. Position the patient on the side that you are not palpating. Have the patient's knee bent on the side you are palpating.

2. Position yourself behind the patient.

3. Palpate with fingers against the abdomen, towards you (posteriorly).

4. The trigger point of the psoas can be found near the ST 25 area, as you gently push your fingers on the abdomen towards you.

5. The trigger point in the iliacus is well hidden and thus difficult to access, although not impossible. It is around the area of GB 28/GB 27, but much more hidden. Try cupping your palm on the iliac crest, and gently push your fingers into the iliacus towards you. Once you find the trigger point, you can gently massage it to deactivate it. This is the safest area for the practitioner to needle if they are not comfortable with deep abdominal needling of the psoas.

6. The trigger point on the inner thigh, where the iliopsoas tendon attaches to the lesser trochanter, can be found by feeling the edge of the pubic bone and the ASIS. The trigger point is about 2 cun down from here, around SP 12.

Caution

The femoral nerve, artery and vein are just below SP 12. Feel for the pulse and needle away from it.

CONCLUDING COMMENTS

The trigger points described here are some of the most common ones that I have come across in my clinical experience that can aggravate pelvic pain in women. Trigger points are more common than we think. Nonetheless it is important and safe practice to first make sure that the pain is not due to an internal organ problem. Besides seeking professional help, there are many self-care skills that patients can use to release their trigger points (see Chapters 8 and 9).

I hope this chapter alerts healthcare professionals as well as women with chronic pelvic pain to the fact that trigger points may be part of the reason for their pain. For healthcare professionals who have never done any deactivating of trigger points, may this chapter stimulate your curiosity to find out more and what to do about them.

CHAPTER 6

FIVE ELEMENTS THEORY-BASED ACUPUNCTURE TREATMENT

INTRODUCTION

The Five Elements theory is important because it provides us with the language and concepts to understand ourselves and others. It originates from ancient Chinese medicine, or Zhong Yi. 'Zhong' means the middle or centre and 'Yi' means oneness, harmony and transformation. The ancient Chinese called this the medicine of the centre, oneness or transformation, and not a medicine of twoness. This is because at its core, it is alchemical or transformational, suggesting there is internal healing and outer changes that reflect our authentic self, the golden flower (Jin Hua), as described in ancient Chinese medical texts.

Acupuncture treatments that are based on the Five Elements theory have provided me with the initial framework, pathway and tool to address my patients' emotional-spiritual health. This approach is crucial because it fills the yawning gap that modern Chinese medicine (traditional Chinese medicine, aka TCM) and biomedicine have largely failed to address. Bridging this gap has become one of the cornerstones of my clinical practice, which is significantly enhanced through incorporating Lorie Eve Dechar's Alchemical Healing and Wang Fengyi's healing approach.[11] Wang Fengyi (born in China in 1864) was an influential healer and preacher who founded a system of Five Elements healing through the emotions. Lorie Eve Dechar is a licensed acupuncturist with a deep grounding in Jungian depth psychology and Taoist alchemy, an author and a teacher, whose approach to healing she has called 'Alchemical Healing'. I have necessarily scratched the surface of this eclectic mix of practices to stimulate your curiosity and interest as well as opening a new way of seeing, being and practising, as these practices have done for me.

The Five Elements are Water, Wood, Fire, Earth and Metal, which are associated with their corresponding organ, season, spirit (Shen), emotion, colour, sound and flavour, as shown in Table 6.1. In health, these elements work together in harmony, like a symphony, with all the musicians playing well together to create a beautiful piece of music. In the Five Elements system, balance and harmony is achieved by each element generating and controlling each other. However, when these dynamics are not working well, there is turmoil and sickness. These different elemental associations enable us to understand human personalities, emotions and consciousness, as this chapter will explore.

Table 6.1. The Five Elements and their associations (influenced by Wang Fengyi's system of Five Elements)

Element	Water	Wood	Fire	Earth	Metal
Organ	Kidney	Liver	Heart	Spleen	Lung
Season	Winter	Spring	Summer	Late Summer	Autumn
Shen (spirit)	Zhi	Hun	Shen	Yi	Po
Emotion	Fear	Anger	Joy	Sympathy	Grief
Emotional poison	Arrogance	Anger	Hate	Blame	Being judgemental
Virtue	Wisdom (Zhi)	Compassion (Ren)	Deep politeness (Li)	Trust/ integrity (Xin)	Selflessness (Yi)
Colour	Black	Green	Red	Yellow	White
Sound	Groan	Shout	Laugh	Sing	Weep

Flavour	Salty	Sour	Bitter	Sweet/bland	Spicy
Power	Storage	Growth	Connection	Harvest	Retreat
Positive qualities	Harmonious and soft (Rou He)	Sense of direction and strategy (Zhu Yi)	Understand sacred connection (Ming Li)	Trust and reliability (Xin Shi)	Clarity (Xiang Liang)
Animal symbol	Turtle and snake	Green dragon	Red bird or phoenix	Yellow bird	White tiger

FIVE ORGANS: THE EXPERIENCE OF EMOTIONS

The movement of Qi (energy) that arises from the five organs is experienced as emotions: fear, anger, joy, sympathy and grief, as associated with the Kidney (Water), Liver (Wood), Heart (Fire), Spleen (Earth) and Lung (Metal), respectively. In Wang Fengyi's healing tradition, negative emotions such as arrogance, anger, hate, blame and being judgemental are called 'emotional poison' because of the potential harm they can inflict. These five organs also respond to the five colours, five sounds and five flavours, as indicated in Table 6.1.

THE FIVE SPIRITS: FIVE STRUCTURES OF CONSCIOUSNESS

Each element is also associated with a spirit: Zhi (Water), Hun (Wood), Shen (Fire), Yi (Earth) and Po (Metal), which can be understood as symbolic representations of psychological functions. These psychic constructs have parallels in the five structures of human consciousness proposed by Jean Gebser (see Johnson 2019). For example, the archaic structure can be said to be related to the Zhi spirit of the Water element, the magical structure to the Po Soul of the Metal element, and the mythical structure to the Hun spirit of the Wood element. Clinically, Gebser's theory provides a crucial theoretical underpinning to understanding the healing energies of the five spirits, which are discussed in the next chapter.

THE FIVE ELEMENTS: PERSONALITY OR TEMPERAMENT

The Five Elements of Water, Wood, Fire, Earth and Metal symbolize the cycle of Qi (energy) in the body throughout the day and night as well as through the seasons. They can be understood as the five temperaments, or personalities. We have all the five personalities within us, but one dominates, a second less so, and the other three play a smaller role. Their clinical importance lies in how these elemental energies enable our patients to understand themselves, and how we, as practitioners, understand the personality of our patients, as well as the most effective way to work with them.

The Five Elements can also be understood as archetypes. They appear repeatedly in stories, paintings or myths across cultures, and enable us to understand our behaviour and how we interact with ourselves and others. Archetypes are symbolic expressions of our innate instinctual energies. They can be our great allies and a guide to our true self when we relate to them appropriately. A good example of an archetype is the earth and fertility goddess, Gaia. In Greek mythology, Gaia is the original source and giver of life and food. Almost all of us have a negative or positive earth archetype within us, which defines the way we relate to ourselves, our bodies, the natural environment and the world. The Swiss psychologist Carl Jung proposed that archetypes live in the deep recess of the human psyche, which he called the 'collective unconscious'. It is in this deep recess of the human psyche that healing takes place, which is thus clinically important and relevant in our work.

THE WATER PERSONALITY: HARMONIOUS AND SOFT

The ancient Chinese believed that Water is the first element because without water there is no life. Although Winter, the season corresponding to Water, comes at the end of the Five Elements cycle, I am presenting it first here because the end also marks the beginning. The Winter season reflects many aspects of the Water personality, such as a preference for solitude, stillness, contemplation, rest, restoration and replenishment. In stillness, the Water personality can contemplate, think deeply and wisely, and tap deep-seated reserves. Water types actively search for intellectual stimulation because its lack makes them unbearably bored. They will spend their energy and time finding a solution to problems and navigating around obstacles rather than engaging in harmful gossip. Like water itself, Water personalities have the capacity and patience to dissolve the hardest of obstacles to achieve what they set out to do.

The Water personality can be destructive when out of balance; they need to be mindful as to how they unleash this energy that destroys anything or anybody that is in their path, just as a tidal wave or tsunami does. Because they pride themselves as someone who can solve problems and achieve, they can be arrogant and dismissive of others. This makes the Water personality unattractive and unbearable. However, when things do not go well, they tend to blame themselves and not others. Their energy is turned inward, and the negative experiences can evolve into helplessness, fearfulness, despair and hopelessness. They become a victim of their negative experience, and when this happens, nothing is achieved.

Emotion and emotional poison: fear and arrogance

Fear is the emotion that is associated with the Water personality, and the emotional poison is arrogance. You will recognize the Water personality when you see a bluish-black tinge to the complexion around the mouth and the laughter lines. When emotionally triggered, this colour goes grey or black. They also have a groaning voice that tends to drop off at the end of a sentence.

The Water personality knows that being fearful can be paralysing, literally like frozen water, and yet it dominates. When in this state, they are unable to be motivated or engaged in any physical or intellectual activity, fearing they may fail to accomplish. This can become a self-fulfilling prophecy. Fear can also swing in the opposite direction, resulting in an apparent disregard for safety, leading them to engage in dangerous activities. Being chronically out of balance can cause the Kidney Qi to weaken and stagnate, resulting in more fear, doubt, anxiety, low back pain and urinary problems. A Water personality needs to truly understand that they can do something about the state of imbalance by transforming fear and arrogance into courage, bravery and wisdom. To undertake transformational work requires cultivating the positive aspects of their personality, and turning their attention inwards to engage in inner work.

The Zhi spirit, the spark that ignites life and instinctual drive

The Zhi spirit is the innate and powerful drive to reproduce, stay alive, achieve and fully blossom, to live the life we are meant to live. It is related to our Source Qi (Yuan Qi), which has the potential power to heal and revitalize. When the Zhi spirit is healthy, the person can be firm and grounded. You will recognize the Zhi spirit is out of balance when there is sleep disturbance, forgetfulness, fear, depression, and lack of initiative, drive or motivation. This person becomes controlling, unable to solve problems or to work towards achieving their goals. There are many causes of a Zhi disturbance, such as overdoing and overexerting to the point of exhaustion, excessive blood loss, traumatic emotional shock, chronic fear and anxiety.

Healing the Water personality

Based on the Wang Fengyi tradition, an out-of-balance Water personality can be recalibrated by the regular practice of self-reflection and turning the light inwards, positively reframing the story we tell ourselves and appealing to the quality of the Water element to transform the emotional poison of being judgemental and fearful into wisdom by daily affirmation and chanting:

> Question: Lao shan ren, gan wo Rou He? [Wise old man, when you see me, am I harmonious and soft?]

> Answer: Wo Rou He! [YES, I am harmonious and soft!]

This affirmation is given as an illustration, which applies to the rest of the four Elements and personalities described later. In working with my patients, however, I do not use this affirmation. Rather, I co-create affirmations with my patients. Further, the process of self-reflection and reframing someone's narrative to a positive one can be adjusted based on the patient's preference, but it must always touch the Heart profoundly for transformation to take place because the Heart is always involved in transformational work, according to Wang Fengyi's healing tradition.

THE WOOD PERSONALITY: SENSE OF DIRECTION AND STRATEGY

Spring is the season that is associated with the Wood element. The stillness of Winter gives way to a flurry of activity. Seedlings and buds push their way into life, defying gravity to reach upwards towards the sun, while the roots fan out and penetrate deeply into the earth for water. Nature presents an image of someone who has a great sense of direction, purpose and drive, and the courage to move forward and to act only when the time is right. Like the branches of a tree or the twisting vine that grows around obstacles, the Wood personality can also overcome impediments and move against the flow to manifest their purpose or vision. Thus, you can be sure that the Wood personality is present whenever there is a new venture. However, all this movement can only happen with the help of the Hun spirit, without which the Wood's purposeful energy and plan will not manifest.

Such characteristics form the blueprint that informs the nature of the Wood personality.

A balanced Wood personality is flexible and can adapt very quickly to changing situations without losing the sense of self. This ability is often likened to the flexibility of the bamboo plant, which bends to whatever direction the wind is blowing, but returns tall and upright when the wind subsides. These types have the potential to accomplish great things and can 'talk the talk and walk the walk', that is, they can put things into action. They can be perceived as attractive to interact with because they talk in a straightforward manner and directly from the heart. When things go wrong, they take responsibility and tend not to put the blame on others.

When Wood personalities exhaust themselves through overwork or stress, they tip out of balance. Consequently, they behave impulsively and rigidly. They are unable to see the big picture or carry out their plan, thus nothing comes to fruition. It can be uncomfortable to be around them because of their rigidity and lack of warmth. When chronically out of balance, the Wood personality shows a tremendous amount of resentment and anger.

Emotion and emotional poison: anger

The Wood personality has the vision to carry out their plan, and needs to find their own path, and live their own vision and dream according to their blueprint. When this energy is persistently and severely stifled, not nurtured or channelled creatively, it turns into resentment and anger. When this happens, the Liver Qi becomes chronically stuck, which manifests in physical symptoms such as bloating, indigestion, irregular menstruation and chronic headaches. The colour around the eyes turns a greenish tinge, the eyes become dull and the body lacks flexibility. Emotionally, this shows up as insomnia, dream-disturbed sleep, irritability and depression.

I find the Chinese character for anger (怒 nù) fascinating and informative. The image depicts a woman with her hands tied behind her back, which also tell us that she has been subjugated. Beneath this image is the radical of the heart. The Chinese character tells us that the creative impulse is not allowed to blossom, transforming the creativity into anger. When this happens, this person can become enslaved by the anger that disrupts and hurts the self and others. The energy of chronic anger can turn inwards and become depression or hopelessness characterized by no impetus, plan or vision to create or start any project, such is the power and force of the frustrated Wood energy. However, when the energy of anger is redirected appropriately, it can be transformed into compassion and love for oneself and for others, as well as the ability to initiate and complete projects.

The Hun spirit, the visionary and dream maker

The Hun spirit is rooted in the Blood of the Liver. The Hun is our Ethereal Soul that comes and goes like the clouds. It is believed that it enters the body shortly after birth, and at death it leaves to return to the heavens. In the daytime, the Hun takes in and processes our daily experiences. At night, the Hun returns to its residence in the Liver to create beneficial dreams and allow restorative sleep. By so doing, the Hun keeps us emotionally balanced. In psychological terms, the Hun is the part of our consciousness that enables us to imagine, to have a vision, a strategy and a direction in life, which is consistent with the internal plan. When that happens, the eyes sparkle with life and energy.

When the Hun is agitated, there is a lack of vitality, vision and direction. Such a person may also be too timid to speak out or start a project, and even if the project is started, it does not come to fruition. They feel stuck, and whichever path they take they feel blocked, which, in turn, makes them more irritable, angry, frustrated and depressed.

Healing the Wood personality

Based on the Wang Fengyi tradition, an out-of-balance Wood personality can be rebalanced by the same methods used for healing the Water personality: regular practice of self-reflection, reframing the story we tell ourselves, and appealing to the positive quality of the Wood to transform the anger and depression into having a plan and a sense of direction (Zhu Yi) by daily affirmation and chanting:

> Question: Lao shan ren, gan wo you Zhu Yi? [Wise old man, when you see me, do I have a plan/vision/direction?]

> Answer: Wo you Zhu Yi! [YES, I have a plan/vision/direction!]

(See the last paragraph in 'Healing the Water personality'.)

THE FIRE PERSONALITY: LOVE AND CONNECTION

The Fire element is associated with the season of Summer when flowers, plants and trees are at the height of their bloom and are stretching out to the sun, as if vying for love and attention. This vitality in the dance of life reflects the spark of awareness and bright consciousness of the Fire personality. Through this spark they reach out to connect, to love with passion, and create intimate relationships that make their life worth living and meaningful. People are attracted to their passion, their ease of connection and the Fire that radiates warmth and passion. Fire types look like they are fun to be with. Thus, the Fire personality often becomes the centre of attention or wants to be the centre of attention. However, the Fire that blazes can also flicker and die out. When that happens, this person can appear cold and passionless.

When the Fire personality is involved in something or with someone else, it is difficult to get their attention because they become intensely focused to the point of losing themselves. They can be vain but may also be full of doubt, and are sometimes deeply concerned about what other people think of them. And yet they think that everyone should look up to them. When the Fire personality is out of balance, they become selfish and have a great sense of entitlement. They become very distrustful of people and suspicious of hidden agendas. They like to talk a lot about making changes in their life because they see that changes are necessary, but it remains just that...talk. According to the teaching of Wang Fengyi, the Fire personality tends to repeat

Emotion and emotional poison: joy and hate

The Heart is associated with the emotion of joy, and hate is the emotional poison. The positive emotion experienced by the Fire personality is deep inner joy or happiness and reverence. To feel joy, the Heart must have experienced bitterness that came from having to endure difficulties and hardships. The colour that is associated with Fire is red, and the taste is bitter. Psychologically, the bitter taste symbolizes that the Fire personality understands that it is important to do the right thing and to follow the right path, even if it is bitter and unpleasant.

When Fire is in balance, there is a right amount of happiness or joy as well as deep reverence for everything in life. When in this state, the Fire personality feels profoundly in rhythm with life and with the beats of the Heart. Consequently, the Fire personality feels the power to transform everything, and their imagination is at its best. Life does not get any better than this!

When the Fire personality is not following its true nature, there is unhappiness, which scatters the spirit and leads to mindless actions that are hurtful. In the extreme, the lack of happiness or joy can manifest as hate, which is a type of lingering and festering anger that, in turn, poisons the Heart. The opposite to hatred is love and a form of deep politeness that springs from sincere reverence for everything. When the hate is not transformed, it poisons the sense of wellbeing, impacting the quality of sleep, and will result in nervousness and anxiety. It is supremely unpleasant to be around someone who is so hateful.

Hate blocks the Qi of the Heart. When the Qi of the Heart (Fire) is blocked, connection with the self, others and the Shen is lost. There are palpitations, restlessness, agitation, dream-disturbed sleep and difficulty falling and staying asleep. The colour around the eyes has a reddish or ash-grey tinge.

The Shen spirit, the Emperor of emotions

The Shen spirit resides in the empty space of the Heart, from which the other four Yin organs derive their power. That might explain why the Heart is called the 'Emperor of emotions'. The Shen is delicate and of utmost importance, and thus must be carefully protected and maintained in its proper place to sustain clarity of mind and consistency in what we say and do. In turmoil, it is important to be still, listen to what our Heart is telling us, and follow the Shen, for it will always show us the right path and direct us to do the right thing. The properly rooted Shen gives us insight, imagination and a strong sense of self.

The red bird is the symbol for the Shen, and it exemplifies its fleeting and delicate nature. You cannot see or touch the Shen, but its presence is reflected in the eyes and the face, which is the flower of the Heart. When our eyes sparkle and our face exudes radiance, the inner vitality of the Shen is comfortably rooted in the empty space of the Heart.

Just like a country that is engaged in civil war and cannot provide a peaceful home for its people, when there is emotional and spiritual agitation, the Heart is no longer able to house the Shen. The face becomes dull, and the eyes are lifeless, as if there is nobody at home. A person with a scattered and homeless Shen has trouble relating to the self and others, and experiences sleep disturbance accompanied by nightmares, deep restlessness and feelings of unrootedness; they are jumpy, and engage in continuous chatter (internally and externally). This person is uncomfortable with silence and experiences anxiety that can culminate in a panic attack. Further, they often express that they no longer feel like themselves and that their life is off track.

Emotional trauma and shock, such as being given a life-threatening diagnosis, physical, emotional or sexual abuse, and other distressing experiences, can cause the Shen to be agitated and leave its dwelling place.

Healing the Fire personality

Based on Wang Fengyi's healing tradition, one of the ways that the Fire personality can help to reconnect with their true nature is by chanting this mantra and affirmation that appeals to the Fire virtue of deep politeness:

Question: Lao shan ren, gan wo Ming Li? [Wise old man, when you see me, do I have sacred connection/understanding?]

Answer: Wo Ming Li! [YES, I have sacred connection/understanding!]

(See the last paragraph in 'Healing the Water personality'.)

THE EARTH PERSONALITY: TRANSFORM, NOURISH AND NURTURE

Like Water, without the Earth there can be no life. The Earth personality is the centre of the Five Elements wheel of life. When the Earth condition is just so, there is the ability to feel what the other is going through with due respect to personal boundaries, and to give the appropriate care and support. The Earth personality is at its best when fully engaged in nourishing and nurturing others as well as themself. They are not only a source of sustenance, but can also shoulder responsibility and persevere, and are not afraid to work hard to bring things to fruition. People feel very comfortable and cared for in the company of an Earth personality. The image is of someone who is soft, fluffy, loving and dependable.

When the Earth personality is out of balance, there is a constant need to give and take care of people, even if it is not wanted. They do not know how to receive, and yet have a deep craving to be nourished and nurtured. When this need is unmet, it leaves them feeling profoundly empty, dissatisfied and discontented, which leads to an inability to accomplish anything. There is a feeling of doing the same thing again and again, being self-obsessed, stuck and frozen in a pattern that retards transformation. Life becomes a challenge and burdensome.

Thus, this person develops a certain hardness and contempt as well as an inability to be touched by the suffering and distress of others.

The colour of the Earth is yellow, which is associated with the colour of the soil or certain grains. In a healthy Earth person, there is a light yellowish around the sides of the eyes, temple and mouth. This colour turns into a deeper yellow when there is a constant need for sympathy and a chronic seeking of nourishment and nurture.

Emotion and emotional poison: sympathy and blame

Showing too much sympathy (too much concern for others at the expense of the self) is a dysfunction that is commonly associated with the Earth personality. They become a crowd pleaser and, in the process, ignore their own needs and then feel contemptuous, resentful and angry. They start to blame others and are unable to take responsibility for their own actions. Chronic blaming and lacking in nourishment eventually manifest as physical symptoms such as bloating, water retention and poor appetite, as well as difficulty focusing and thinking clearly, forgetfulness and overthinking things.

The Earth personality should be aware that blame can be transformed into trust in the self and others, having integrity and the ability to set boundaries as well as take responsibility for what they say and do.

The Yi spirit, action reflecting words

The Yi spirit resides in the Spleen. The Yi gives us the ability to focus the mind, process ideas and organize thoughts. A healthy Yi speaks from the Heart so that actions reflect our words or desires, and it also supports us in digesting and assimilating our psycho-emotional experience. The Yi is often translated to mean 'intention', and healthy intention helps ideas, plans or living things manifest at the appropriate time. The Yi reflects the insight of the Shen, manifests the grand vision of the Hun, helps the Po to feel and see clearly, and carries out the Zhi's drive to become. The Yi spirit is essential, as without it nothing can manifest.

When the Yi is out of balance, it is not surprising that ideas or plans do not get completed. An unhealthy Yi is unable to speak from the Heart, and the person's actions are not consistent with their words or desires. Energy is used up in obsessive thoughts, worry and overthinking, and always needing to please others out of a sense of neediness. When the neediness is not met, it is easy to turn to food for comfort, and a poor relationship with food can develop.

Healing the Earth personality

Based on Wang Fengyi's healing tradition, one of the ways that the Earth personality can help to reconnect with the authentic self is to appeal to the positive qualities by chanting this mantra and affirmation, which appeals to the Earth virtue of trust and integrity:

Question: Lao shan ren, gan wo Xin Shi? [Wise old man, when you see me, do I have trust/integrity?]

Answer: Wo Xin Shi! [YES, I have trust/integrity!]

(See the last paragraph in 'Healing the Water personality'.)

THE METAL PERSONALITY: LOGICAL AND PRECISE

Metal in Chinese means gold (Jin). Metal is associated with Autumn, when the trees and plants shed their golden-brown leaves. This foliage forms layers on the soil, and as it decays and rots, it enriches the soil that will, in turn, provide nutrients to the seeds, seedlings and maturing plants. I believe that it is the life-sustaining nutrients that come from the decaying foliage that are being referred to as Jin. Like the decaying foliage that enriches the soil, the Metal personality is selfless and charitable, and performs deeds for the common good. They are logical and precise in their thoughts, and execute plans in great detail. They are not secretive and their actions are transparent. They have extremely high standards in their personal and professional life, and hold others to the same standards. This is a double-edged sword, however, and can pose a problem for the Metal personality.

When out of balance, the Metal personality becomes judgemental and stuck in the minutiae of life, which can be unproductive. At their very worst, they are prone to jealousy and like to engage in negative talks about others. Their actions and words can turn vengeful and hurtful. However, they will always be able to justify to themselves that their hurtful action is acceptable, even it is not, but nonetheless they are likely to have a sense of guilt and regret.

Emotion and emotional poison: grief and being judgemental
Grief, if not processed appropriately, can lodge in the body for a long time, create stagnation and weaken the lungs. [AQ] When the Qi of the Lungs (Metal) is stagnated, there will be problems with the respiratory system such as asthma and a cough. If chronically out of balance, the Metal personality feels depressed, restless and anxious, and becomes hypersensitive, selfish and stingy.

The emotional poison for the Metal personality is being judgemental and highly critical of everything and everybody. Because they are unable to accept and let go, they feel stifled and unable to create a pathway and space for new possibilities. But if they learn to be less judgemental and hypercritical, they can regain their virtue of selflessness to become an invaluable member of society. The Metal personality needs to know and learn that grief and judgement can be transformed into selflessness and generosity in thoughts and actions.

The Po Soul, our body knowing
The Lung is the residence of the Po Soul. While the Hun is ethereal and celestial, the Po Soul is firmly rooted in the physical reality of the body. It is believed that at death the Po Soul disintegrates and returns to the earth. According to Lorie Eve Dechar, the Po Soul plays an important role in Alchemical Healing and transformation because it is an invaluable source of our deep instinctual knowing at the level of our body. In health, the Po Soul responds to the Lung and Large Intestine to facilitate our deep instinctual knowing, or our 'gut feeling'. When we are deeply grounded in our body, we can take in what is nourishing

and let go of what is not. Because the Po Soul largely depends on the health of the Hun and the Shen, the Po Soul gets agitated when these are out of balance. An agitated Po Soul becomes self-destructive in the form of addictions and compulsions.

Healing the Metal personality

Based on Wang Fengyi's tradition, an out-of-balance Metal personality can be recalibrated by the regular practice of self-reflection, reframing the story we tell ourselves and appealing to the positive quality of the Metal to transform the emotional poison of being judgemental by daily affirmation and chanting:

> Question: Lao shan ren, gan wo Xiang Liang? [Wise old man, when you see me, do I have radiance of sound and light?]
>
> Answer: Wo Xiang Liang! [YES, I have radiance of sound and light!]

Xiang Liang is translated to mean a voice that is loud and clear, that is, having clarity in our thoughts and judgement.

(See the last paragraph in 'Healing the Water personality'.)

FIVE ELEMENTS-STYLE ACUPUNCTURE TREATMENT

It was the well-respected British acupuncturist J.R. Worsley (1923–2003) who popularized Five Elements acupuncture in the West. Its premise is in diagnosing the one element that is the cause and source of imbalance in the patient. Accordingly, the primary goal is to address that imbalance, and to return the patient to harmony. The diagnosis of the elemental imbalance is based on the patient's presenting signs, such as the colour of the face, sound of the voice, odour and display of inappropriate emotions rather than physical symptoms, such as pain and sleep disturbances. Accordingly, treatment is aimed at correcting the element that is most out of balance, with the emphasis on the emotional-spiritual health. I have adopted aspects of this style of Five Elements acupuncture into my clinical practice.

Other approaches that I have integrated into my clinical practice are primarily from Lorie Eve Dechar's Alchemical Healing and Dr Tan's Balance Method (BM), depending on the patient's most pressing health concerns. Obviously, since most of my patients experience severe pelvic pain that has its origin in an organic cause such as endometriosis, the BM is the treatment of choice. Having said that, it is important to note that our physical health is intimately linked to our psycho-emotional-spiritual health. It is almost impossible to separate these entities. Thus, in every instance it is crucial to assess the patient carefully and comprehensively.

THE FIVE ELEMENTS TREATMENT PROTOCOLS

The Five Elements unblocking acupuncture treatment protocols that I use are the Aggressive Energy, Internal Dragons and External Dragons treatments, which are rather mysterious sounding and even bordering on the supernatural. However, it is important to understand that these treatments are deeply rooted in the very heart of ancient Chinese medicine. It is equally important to be able to explain in understandable lay terms what these treatments entail and what they aim to achieve, which is to return the patient to a state of health and harmony.

Aggressive Energy treatment

Aggressive energy or 'Xie' Qi (evil Qi (energy)) can be internally or externally generated and is considered one of the several energetic blocks to healing. Xie Qi can be externally generated by conditions such as dry, damp, heat and cold. Patients who are chronically exposed to these conditions can succumb to them, especially if their health is somewhat compromised, making them internally vulnerable. Xie Qi is also often present when there is trauma, shock and chronic emotional dissonance.

Many, but not all, the patients I've treated tend to present with both externally and internally generated Xie Qi. My patient population suffers from chronic pain, which is a source of enormous stress as well as emotional and psychological turmoil. Often, these conditions translate into loss of a sense of self and relationship problems with the self and significant others as well as in social or work relationships (Chong *et al.* 2018a). These internally generated problems can cause the Qi to stagnate, and then to invade and dwell in the internal organs. Patients may have signs and symptoms that are associated with the elemental emotions and emotional poisons such as anger, a sense of hatred, blame, inability to process grief, in addition to experiencing fear, anxiety, depression, exhaustion, panic attacks and disturbed sleep. When these symptoms are present together with a pulse that has a superficial or deep 'vibrational' quality (a quivering feel), I know that the Aggressive Energy treatment is indicated.

PREPARING THE PATIENT

In explaining to patients about the Aggressive Energy treatment, I seldom use the term 'aggressive energy', but instead I say a few sentences to this effect:

> There is energy in your body that does not serve you. This treatment aims to unblock this energy by putting needles superficially on your back so that you can enjoy a sense of wellbeing.
>
> Most patients report a sense of calmness after the treatment. However, it is important to be aware that everyone is different. Listen to your bodily sensations and emotions and accept what comes up. You may wish to keep a journal to record your experience.

NEEDLING TECHNIQUE

I always use a guide tube to control the depth of the needles. Gently tap the needles to just below the surface of the skin so that they flop over when in position. There is no need to manipulate or push the needles deeper. Patients are treated in a prone position or seated on a chair with their back facing the practitioner. I usually use 0.20 x 40mm needles. Aggressive Energy treatment is an excellent first treatment for patients who have never had acupuncture before, as it is gentle and relaxing as well as effective.

POINTS USED IN AGGRESSIVE ENERGY TREATMENT: BACK SHU POINTS

Back Shu points provide a conduit between them and the organs they serve. These points are located on the inner bladder line, midway between the centre of the spine and the inner edge of the scapula. Points are needled bilaterally, from top to bottom and right to left:

- UB (UB) 13 (back Shu of the Lung)

- UB 14 (back Shu of the Heart Protector/Pericardium)

- UB 15 (back Shu of the Heart)

- UB 18 (back Shu of the Liver)

- UB 20 (back Shu of the Spleen)

- UB 23 (back Shu of the Kidney).

HOW TO TELL IF AGGRESSIVE ENERGY IS PRESENT

If aggressive energy is present, a circle of redness generally gathers around the needles; the needles are not removed until the redness has dissipated. This may take a few minutes or much longer. If the redness is still present after 45–60 minutes, take the needles out and repeat the treatment at the next visit.

WATCHING OUT FOR THE HEART

Because the Heart houses the Shen, which is very sensitive, UB 15 (Heart) is not needled until all the other points have been fully drained of aggressive energy. Sometimes it takes several repetitions of Aggressive Energy treatment before all the aggressive energy is cleared, and before the Heart can be needled, as in the case of my patient presented later in this chapter. Generally, the needle is not retained when needling UB 15.

PULSE

Always check the patient's pulse before needle insertions, and recheck during treatment and after the needles have been removed to ensure that the pulse has been harmonized. When that happens, the pulse position's cun (first position from the wrist), Guan (middle position) and Chi (third position) feel calmer and more balanced. This harmonization is also reflected in the patient's eyes and colour of the face.

Clearing possession: Internal and External Dragons treatment

Another energetic block to healing is possession, which blocks the Heart (the Emperor) from sensing, seeing and hearing clearly. When this happens, the patient is no longer in full possession of their faculties, and they often report feeling 'strange'; they no longer feel like themselves. Possession can be caused by extreme temperature fluctuations, drugs, a serious accident, emotional betrayal, a terrifying experience such as emotional shock due to the sudden death of a loved one, or vulnerability due to incest or abuse. The eyes, being the windows of the soul, give the cardinal signs of possession: the patient has a vacant look and hooded eyes, and difficulty making eye contact for a sustained time. This patient is often not quite present. Clinically, I often feel like I have not been able to reach them, and somehow the encounter feels incomplete and unsatisfactory.

The two treatments for clearing possession are called the 'Seven Dragons treatment'. These are the Internal Dragons and External Dragons treatments. In Chinese medicine and culture, the mythical dragons are good, powerful and benevolent. These two treatments are meant to summon the benevolent heavenly dragons to dislodge the demons that are in possession of the Heart, so that the Shen can return to its rightful home, and we can be ourselves again. My patients often find these descriptions of dragons and demons useful images to have as part of their imagery exercises.

Internal Dragons treatment

The Internal Dragons treatment is appropriate in extreme situations of psycho-emotional shock as in the sudden death of a loved one, an unwanted and unanticipated divorce with emotional betrayal, vulnerability due to incest or abuse, being chronically sleep-deprived, exhaustion because of extreme hard work and an inability to replenish oneself.

POINTS NEEDLED

- ¼ inch below Ren 15 (Conception Vessel)
- ST 25 (bilateral)
- ST 32 (bilateral)
- ST 41 (bilateral)
- For depression, replace ST 25 with a point halfway between ST 36 and ST 37.

External Dragons treatment

External Dragons treatment is indicated when the underlying cause comes from outside events such as being involved in a road traffic accident, addiction to drugs or alcohol or prolonged and severe exposure to either extreme heat or extreme cold.

POINTS NEEDLED

- DU 20
- UB 11 (bilateral)
- UB 23 (bilateral)
- UB 61 (bilateral).

NEEDLING TECHNIQUE

Needles are inserted from right to left, top to bottom, with a 360-degree counter-clockwise turn to disperse the unwanted evil Qi. Needles are left for 20–30 minutes until the pulses have harmonized or contact with the patient is easier. Depth of needle insertion is no more than 0.5 cun and against the flow of Qi. It is important that the patient experiences the Qi sensation.

DID THE TREATMENT WORK?

You know that the treatment has worked when you see a calmer patient, a more radiant face and eyes that are brighter and able to make eye contact easier. I often inform my patients to be more aware of the comings and goings of their emotions. Some patients may respond by crying or feeling sad. Whatever the treatment response(s) might be, I suggest that they go with the flow and make space for them.

CASE STUDY

A young lady was referred to me for depression, anxiety, disturbed sleep and not feeling rested in the morning. She was crying a lot, and often said that she did not know what had happened to her as she did not recognize or feel like herself any more. This immediately made me realize that her Shen was agitated. She was diagnosed with endometriosis and had had pelvic pain for many years. Her pulse was thin and had a chaotic quality to it. Her tongue had a thick yellow coat, and was redder at the sides and tip. Prickles were observed, especially at the tip of the tongue.

She maintained little eye contact during the first consultation. As she recounted her journey from having pain at 12 years old when she started her period to her diagnosis at age 22, her face turned a deep greenish colour around the eyes and mouth areas, which gave me an inkling that her Wood element was also in disharmony. She was very angry and upset.

I gave her an Aggressive Energy treatment, after having explained to her what this treatment entailed, as described earlier. After the needles were inserted, I noticed a significant amount of aggressive energy was present. These circles of redness were so large that they overlapped one another. She received two more treatments before the aggressive energy was drained satisfactorily. She reported that after her first treatment she felt much calmer, restored and rested in the morning.

Once the aggressive energy had been drained, she received an Internal Dragons treatment, an External Dragons treatment, and then another Aggressive Energy treatment on consecutive subsequent visits.

I followed up with an Internal Dragons and an External Dragons treatment because of her depression and anxiety, but significantly she had very little eye contact with me at the beginning. In more serious cases, the spark and twinkle in the eyes are replaced by a vacant look. Further, she had reported that she felt that she did not recognize herself, or did not feel like herself any more. These, to me, are indicative of a disturbed and agitated Shen, the spirit of the Heart. The agitation had invaded deep into and overtaken the Heart space so that she was no longer in control of her faculties.

After these treatments, she began to feel more in charge of herself. Her sleep was much improved, and she felt significantly less anxious. We agreed the next steps would be to work on the issue of anger and to address the endometriosis-associated pain using the Balance Method. Although this description gives the impression that I am separating the physical from the psycho-emotional treatment, in reality these two are opposite sides of the same coin. Thus, over many months I integrated many of the Alchemical Healing tools and skills into her overall care.

CONCLUDING THOUGHTS
How does transformation happen?

In this chapter I have introduced the Five Elements theory, the emotions, spirits and personalities as well as a case study to highlight how I used the theory and the treatment protocols.

The essence of ancient Chinese medicine (Zhong Yi) is

transformation and the return of the person to their wholeness. Can this happen by merely mastering the Aggressive Energy, Internal Dragons and External Dragons protocols? The answer is no. Anyone can be taught to do these protocols, but to initiate the healing process and bring about transformation requires the integration of other skills. In my clinical practice, the treatments are invaluable as a starting point for many of my patients' healing process. Transformation happens with deep inner work on our emotional chaos, turmoil and struggles that result in inner and outer changes. This kind of deep work is very challenging, and it requires patience and the ability to hold the space for discomfort during the process. This is where Alchemical Healing comes in, which is the subject of the next chapter.

FURTHER READING

Dechar, L.E. (2006) *Five Spirits: Alchemical Acupuncture for Psychological and Spiritual Healing*. New York: Lantern Books.

Dechar, L.E. (2021) *Kigo: Exploring the Spiritual Essence of Acupuncture Points through the Changing Seasons*. London: Singing Dragon.

Dechar, L.E. and Fox, B. (2021) *The Alchemy of Inner Work: A Guide for Turning Illness & Suffering into True Health & Well-Being*. Newburyport, MA: Red Wheel/Weiser.

Fruehauf, H. (2009) 'All disease comes from the heart: The pivotal role of the emotions in Classical Chinese medicine.' https://classicalchinesemedicine. org/all-disease-comes-from-heart-pivotal-role-emotions-classical-chinese-medicine

Hicks, A., Hicks, J. and Mole, P. (2004) *Five Element Constitutional Acupuncture*. Edinburgh, London, New York: Churchill Livingstone.

Jarrett, L.S. (2006) *The Clinical Practice of Chinese Medicine*. Stockbridge, MA: Spirit Path Press.

Larre, C. and Rochat de la Vallée, E. (1995) *Rooted in Spirit: The Heart of Chinese Medicine*. Barrytown, NY: Station Hill Press.

—— CHAPTER 7 ——

AN ALCHEMICAL HEALING APPROACH TO TRANSFORMING PSYCHO-EMOTIONAL DISTRESS

INTRODUCTION

As alluded to in the previous chapter, this chapter is about working with a patient's psycho-emotional pain. This kind of work necessarily goes beyond treating the physical body, which provides a container for healing and transformation to occur. It calls for a healing relationship that is co-created with the active participation of the patient and the practitioner. This aspect of my work is much influenced by Lorie Eve Dechar's Alchemical Healing (Dechar and Fox 2021), which uses different tools to move the patient's Qi and touch their soul. These tools could include the spiritual meaning of acupuncture points, acupuncture needling, Breathwork, rituals, Inner Sensing, active imagination, and the use of flower essences and essential oils.

Healing in this context is focused on nurturing life and supporting a person's return to wholeness or the authentic self. Alchemy is the 'art and science of transformation' (Dechar and Fox 2021, p.7), which results in an enhanced inner and outer self. Over the many years that I've studied with Lorie Eve Dechar, I have adapted the Alchemical Healing skills and tools specifically for my patient population.[12]

For many years I did not have the theoretical framework to articulate satisfactorily to myself or to patients how or why some of the Alchemical Healing tools are therapeutic. Jean Gebser's theory of consciousness provided me with what I have been searching for (see Johnson 2019). Gebser proposed five structures of consciousness – archaic, magical, mythical, mental and integral – which I find incredibly useful. In this chapter, I have presented two patient examples to highlight the use of some of the Alchemical Healing tools and ways of accessing the healing energies from the archaic, magical and mythical structures. These are interwoven, for confidentiality reasons, from a composite profile derived from my US and UK patients.

PATIENT NO. 1, HEALING PSYCHIC AND EMOTIONAL PAIN

This 40-year-old woman was no longer responding to conventional approaches to her chronic pelvic pain. She had been consulting with a psychiatrist for anxiety and depression, but was adamant that she did not want or need any medications. I thought this was most unusual as in my experience most patients tend to want to treat these problems with medications, perhaps not realizing that there are other ways. This led me to a fleeting thought that she had a very good insight into her anxiety and depression. On further reflection, I suspected that she knew deep down that she could not medicate herself out of her problems. What I did not know then was the depth of her despair.

At our initial visit, I saw an exhausted woman, but the most striking feature was her eyes. They had lost their vital sparkle and shine, which told me that the Shen, the very essence of the self and soul, was not firmly rooted in the Heart space. In fact, her eyes were dull, lifeless and hollow. Her face lacked vitality and her voice was flat. I took a few deep breaths and carefully noted my bodily sensations. I felt her emotional turmoil and her effort to keep it under control. A sadness and a kind of hollowness surrounded me. I saw a lost and fearful young child who was desperately looking for her way 'home'.

She recounted a life filled with fear, anxiety, anger and emptiness, and a total lack of joy and happiness. She did not see the point in living, but had never contemplated suicide. She had disturbed sleep with vivid nightmares, and thus never or seldom experienced the velvety feeling of a restorative good night's sleep. She shifted uncomfortably in her seat and then looked away as she talked about how, for the longest time, she had felt deep shame, guilt and unworthiness. I initially felt a lot of sadness, but as I listened, in this sadness I saw an optimistic horizon. I firmly believed that she had the power within her to do the necessary transformational work. Despite being disconnected with her authentic self and her Shen being agitated, hidden deep down I saw a tiny spark of steely and undaunted determination. Many months later, and after many hours of hard work, I was to witness the growing of this tiny spark and the unfurling of this determination. We both knew that the journey ahead of us was going to be challenging. We talked at length about the process of working together, and she understood that it was through adversity that movement, growth and healing could happen. We agreed to our lengthy collaboration to mend and recover the lost self with various tools such as Inner Sensing, Breathwork, visualization and Five Elements acupuncture (see Chapter 6).

Initial acupuncture treatment

Over the course of several visits, she received the three Five Elements acupuncture treatments to clear contaminated energy that was obstructing the free flow of Qi (energy) (see the section in Chapter 6 on Aggressive Energy, Internal Dragons and External Dragons). The Aggressive Energy treatment was repeated several times until almost all the erythema (redness) had been cleared from the needled points on her back. At different treatment sessions, I also added the outer back Shu point such as UB 42 Po Hu (Door of the Corporal Soul) (Deadman, Al-Khafaji and Baker 2001), to support her grieving process, and UB 52 Zhi Shi (Ambition Room), to help her find strength in her search for her authentic self (Dechar 2021). Needling these points did not mean that such goals were realized; rather, it was the recruitment of the narrative of the acupuncture points, imagery and the setting of an intention for the treatment that really made a difference.

Breathwork and visualization: 'Invitation to Return Home'

When she was ready, I taught her the Breathwork and visualization 'Invitation to Return Home' (presented in Chapter 1) to use during the acupuncture treatments or when she was at home. In her visualization, the image she needed to create was a little red bird, the mythical bird associated with the Shen. Like most of my patients, she initially had difficulty visualizing the image. After several attempts, the image came. She was able to describe the bird, which for her was neither white nor red, but purple. She found the purple bird sitting on her shoulder chirping away! She was very excited about the appearance of her purple bird. Once she had the image, she gently invited it back to her Heart space. However, there were times when she could not see the image of the bird, only total darkness and a terrifying kind of emptiness and fear. But, with time and perseverance, she learned not to fight the fear, to breathe through it and stay with it, and recruited her 'felt sense' (see 'Inner Sensing: a magical structure experience' later in this chapter) into her imagery and breathing exercise. She became quite good at it and found the combination helpful.

The golden key

In the many months that followed, and on my suggestion, she kept a journal to record her thoughts, emotions, or any events that seemed significant to her. Gradually, a pattern emerged. After each treatment, she would feel better, and by the time she returned for another treatment, she had relapsed. She was beginning to feel somewhat despondent, and I was puzzled as to why she was not making any sustained progress. I reminded myself of the Alchemical Healing notion of sitting with the discomfort, of not knowing and to follow what my heart was telling me. Then, one day I had the 'Aha' moment as I was just daydreaming.

I felt this unmistakable bodily sensation that I had missed something fundamental and crucial to her healing. At that very 'Aha' moment I received the golden key to her suffering. It was the deep shame, guilt and unworthiness that she had mentioned at our first meeting. I suspected that these feelings of shame and guilt had their roots in being traumatized in her childhood, but I felt it was not the right time to initiate this conversation until she was ready to do so.

One day she came in sobbing, looking very distressed and exhausted. I did not know what to do as there was not much I could do, except to be present, compassionate and kind as she cried. This expression of pain went on for what seemed like a long time until she was ready to talk. She told a story of being abused as a young child. She had kept this a big secret because she felt profoundly ashamed, unworthy and guilty – ashamed and guilty because she felt that she had caused the abuse and thus deserved it. Dealing with her chronic pain had triggered the deeply buried traumatic experience, which she had hoped she had banished for life by making a conscious effort not to remember or acknowledge its presence. I felt a physical ache in my heart as I listened to her story. I saw this terrified and lost young child, unanchored and untethered in what seemed like a cruel and uncaring world. What she needed most was love and kindness. My work was to help her recover the lost self and soul, and to feel safety in the knowledge that out of the broken pieces a whole could and would emerge. In the subsequent acupuncture treatments, I asked her to imagine nurturing and to hold her own inner child, that young girl, with love.

The spirit and healing power of acupuncture point names

After she had finished crying, we discussed how to help her to open up a little in a way that did not feel threatening, to let in some inner peace and calmness. Setting my intention to align with the spirit of the point, I gently needled PC 6 Nei Guan (Inner Gate), located 2 inches above the transverse crease of the wrist, between the two tendons of the palmaris longus and flexor carpi radialis muscles. This point is excellent for calming a restless heart and stilling a busy mind agitated by trauma and its ramifications. I also reminded my patient to practise the Breathwork and visualization 'Invitation to Return Home', inviting her purple bird routine, and to imagine receiving the peace and calmness into her real authentic self. I repeated this treatment as needed.

Subsequent treatments also included other points such as the upper Kidney points, which my patient found very meaningful and empowering: KI 24 Ling Xu (Spirit Burial Ground) and KI 25 Shen Cang (Spirit Storehouse), both located on the upper Kidney meridian, on the third and second intercostal space, respectively, two fingers from the midline. KI 24 aims to restore spiritual strength, which would aid in the recovery of the soul and her true self. Kidney 25 promotes healing at times of distress and suffering due to betrayal and profound loss. KI 25, like a storehouse, has the inner resources that she could draw on any time.[13] These points were needled with care and gentleness, with no stimulation. I also suggested that she visualize and breathe into UB 52 Zhi Shi (Ambition Room). UB 52 is 3 cun lateral to DU 4 at the level of the spinous process of the 2nd lumbar vertebra. This is known as the Mingmen (The Gate of Life or Vitality) in Chinese medicine or in Alchemical Healing, and it is likened to the space where Gebser's archaic structure is situated, both of which are our source of healing energies. The Taoists believe that this point supports the drive or ambition to become *me*.

Ritual

In working with her, I recalled my family's practice of showing respect and love and reconnecting with the souls of our ancestry at the altar of worship, placed in a prominent area of our home. We offer this practice with a simple ritual of burning incense in the morning and evening. Following this session, she built her own altar and created a ritual to love and nurture the inner child in her and to 'interact' with her family, whom she felt had failed her. She reported that during this ritual she experienced a deep warm feeling in her chest area, and felt that she was reclaiming herself.

Darkness into light

During our sessions together and in her dreams, one of the most enduring and recurrent images she saw was her young self in a deep and pitch-dark well. All her efforts to climb out of the well were futile and she could only see black and darkness. In her sleep, she would jump up in a panic. Gradually, over time and after many treatment sessions, the darkness gave way to a little patch of blue sky, then a bigger patch, until it grew to be a complete whole. We both knew then that she could and would climb out of that deep well and step into the power of herself. Gradually, her psycho-emotional pain subsided, even if it did not totally disappear. However, importantly, and when necessary, she now had the skills and tools to work with.

PATIENT NO. 2, ALCHEMY OF TURNING FEAR AND ANGER INTO WISDOM AND COMPASSION

This 40-year-old woman suffered from severe chronic pelvic pain with long-standing deep fear and suppressed anger. She also had a history of breast cancer, which had been treated successfully. She was a very accomplished woman with a successful business, but hated her job and her life. She was not living the life that she was meant to live. When we first met, she was unable or maybe not ready to articulate her emotional state. She had dark rings around her eyes, which gave her a haunted look. She had recurrent nightmares and disturbed sleep, and did not feel rested in the morning. In fact, she was chronically tired. Her most distinguishing feature was her inability to get in touch with her emotions, and she therefore did not even know what emotions she had, much less express them. She found it difficult to engage in Inner Sensing or visualization, but was able to follow simple instructions to do some simple breath-in and breath-out. As I scanned my own bodily sensations, I came up with a lot of confusion, and I really did not have a definite plan as to how to proceed. But I stayed with the confusion and did not try to do anything with it, trusting that she would talk when she was ready to do so. I also trusted that my own intuition would lead me to do the right thing. And indeed, one day something shifted in the most unexpected manner.

As usual, she did not much want to engage in conversation and responded to my questions in monosyllabic answers. I respected her need to be silent. And I reminded myself to stay with my discomfort of not knowing. She followed my instructions to place one hand on the heart area and the other on the lower dantian (the area between the belly button and the pubic bone), to imagine dropping into the lower dantian with each breath-in and breath-out, a form of embodied centring using Breathwork. I reminded her to always return to this breathing exercise when life became too unbearable and chaotic.

The benevolent dragon

I invited her and she agreed to evoke the image of the dragon to help her in whatever ways she felt she needed help when she was receiving an Internal Dragons treatment. I explained to her that in Chinese medicine, the dragon symbolizes strength, wisdom, benevolence and knowledge. I had just completed the needle insertions when I noticed her body was shaking. I realized that she was sobbing quietly and was trying to suppress it. It seemed like the more she tried to suppress the sobbing, the stronger her body shook. I proceeded to remove the needles. She sat up and this time she let out a loud sob. I was alarmed, and my first thought was that the image of the dragon had scared her, but then I realized that this was her 'Aha' moment. I noticed the sides of her eyes, temples and around the mouth had turned a dark green with distinct tinges of black. Normally, I would not interrupt this very private moment, but I felt that it was appropriate for me to do so because my intuition informed me that this was fundamental to her healing process. I saw a tiny crack with a beam of light shining through, and was hopeful that this might start the process of getting in touch with her emotions.

I gave her a small mirror so that she could look at the colour of her face. The second she saw the colour, she stopped crying. She was curious as to what it all meant. I explained that the colour green was related to anger (Wood), and black to fear (Water). I suggested to her that perhaps these were the emotions that she was experiencing but had been unable to access or describe. These emotions, I added, could be transformed into courage and compassion, first and foremost for herself and then for others. I could see this resonated deeply with her. Her need to talk burst open like the sluice gate that had been dammed up over many years. She was very unhappy in her marriage, specifically, and with life in general. She was very angry with her husband, whom she felt had let her down. She also had a deep fear of being abandoned and left alone to cope with her children. She had wanted to leave her husband for a long time and yet had never had the courage to do so. This time she cried freely as she told her story. When she left, she looked emotionally drained but calm. She murmured a 'Thank you'.

Needling KI 1 Yong Guan (Bubbling Spring)

I explained to her the meaning of the acupuncture point named KI 1 Yong Guan (Bubbling Spring). I chose this point because it would ground and centre her, calm the Shen and allow her suppressed anger to bubble out. KI 1 conjures up energy that is bubbling and bursting forth. I instructed her to take a few breaths in and out, and to lower her eyelids while I placed my thumbs on the soles of her feet, about two-thirds from the heel. She began to relax. As usual I set my intention to reflect the spirit of the point, and as soon as the needles were inserted, she gave a deep sigh and her breathing slowed down.

She left with a little twinkle in her eyes and stated that the huge weight that she had been carrying for years had been lifted. This was the inflection point as I could feel a shift in her and in our relationship. I knew that in our next sessions she would be open to learning how to be in touch with her bodily sensations through Inner Sensing, which we did in several of our sessions. Over time, she became very good at the process and was able to articulate her bodily sensations, and to name the emotions associated with the sensations in our subsequent sessions. I was confident that she was going to do something about her situation, which would mark the beginning of her healing and transformational journey.

THE CLINICAL SIGNIFICANCE OF GEBSER'S STRUCTURES OF CONSCIOUSNESS

I feel it is important and essential to give voice, however brief, to Gebser's theory of consciousness. This is because of its clinical significance in providing an enlightening frame of reference for the Alchemical Healing tools that I used for my two patients and in my clinical practice. Gebser's theory of consciousness relates to the archaic, mental, magical, mythical and integral structures. However, for the purpose of this chapter, I have focused on the different ways to efficiently access the latent healing energies of the archaic, magical and mythical structures (Table 7.1) (Dechar, Fox and Shaw 2020).

Table 7.1. Efficient ways to access the archaic, magical and mythical structures

Archaic structure Connecting with the Original Source	Acupuncture, e.g., Aggressive Energy treatment Cranial sacral therapy Chanting Embodied centring with Breathwork Listening to music Meditation Reiki Shaking Qigong Visualization or imagery Yoga Zero balancing
Magical structure Listening deeply to gut feelings, smells, sounds	Acupuncture (release emotional block) Affirmations (positive) Deep listening Inner Sensing Meditation with Breathwork Ritual healing Rhythm and dancing Prayer Setting an intention

Mythical structure	Archetypes
Heart-centred knowing	Heart-centred Meditation
	Holding the space in discomfort (Wu Wei)
	Imagination
	Re-telling our life's stories
	Spirits of acupuncture points

The dominant mental structure

The most impactful of the mental structure is the development of an ego and the ability to have a point of view. We humans pride ourselves as thinking and rational beings with the ability to understand ideas, digest them and solve complex problems. Thus, logical human thought has provided the foundation and shaped modern Western science and medicine, which we have benefited from enormously. However, the deficient use of the mental structure shows up in the dualistic nature of modern Western medicine with its primary focus on the body at the cost of excluding the soul and spirit-based therapies that are not deemed 'evidence-based medicine' and cannot be logically explained. Consequently, we are left with a very narrow, sterile and unsatisfactory definition of health based largely on the lack of physical diseases. This way of thinking about health primarily defines and heavily dominates how healthcare is conceived and delivered.

As the mental structure becomes increasingly dominant, there is a push-back against its hegemony to create something more inclusive and meaningful for our complicated and multidimensional health problems. To that end, the call is to remember, recognize and activate the forgotten and latent healing energies of the archaic, magical and mythical structures so that we can be fully engaged and integrated (the manifestation of the integral structure). Alchemical Healing believes that inherent in these structures are energies that we can tap into to heal ourselves.

Healing energies of the archaic structure

The clinical significance of the archaic structure is its healing potential, especially in treating patients who have suffered from traumatic events, fear and feelings of hopelessness. The archaic structure comes from a primordial presence that springs into time. In Alchemical Healing, the archaic structure is said to be associated with the Water element, where our powerful and revitalizing Source Qi (original Qi) resides. Its physical space can be located at the lower dantian (the area between the navel and the pubic bone). It has its resonance with the Taoist idea of our unadulterated original nature (authentic self) where the self (ego) has yet to develop, that is, before we are aware of ourselves as a separate entity.

There are many ways to efficiently tap into these healing energies, such as acupuncture, cranial sacral therapy, Reiki, chanting, Shaking Qigong, Yoga, embodied centring using Breathwork to access the lower dantian, Meditation, visualization and listening to music. In the clinical healing space, when the practitioner can simultaneously hold the space between two opposing and uncomfortable situations, yet be able to stay present with themselves and the patient, the spontaneous and unexpected new possibility for healing can emerge from the archaic source.

Magical structure: what does my gut feeling want me to know?

Magical consciousness is about being in touch with and trusting our bodily sensations when we enquire, 'What does my gut feeling want me to know?' Its central therapeutic application is in connecting with and listening deeply to the messages of our gut feeling (intuition), and to intuitively know what needs to be heard. This body-knowing facilitates visceral connection where no words are needed as healing comes from the energetic exchanges between two people. Magical consciousness invites an Alchemical Healing practice that enables the practitioner to be steadfastly present with the patient, aligning themselves both to what is happening in the treatment room as well as to the field of relationship between them and their patient, while also maintaining a healthy boundary in order not to be lost in the patient's suffering.

Setting an intention to a treatment, Inner Sensing, ritual healing, rhythmic chants, positive affirmations, dance or movement and listening to the gut feeling are examples of enrolling the power of the magical structure. The Five Elements acupuncture treatment for releasing emotional-spiritual blocks that hinder deep bodily knowing is another example of accessing the energies of the magical structure.

Mythical structure: what does my heart want me to know?

In the mythical structure the knowing comes from the heart, and consciousness begins to evolve into a higher state of self-awareness. Along with this heightened awareness comes the understanding of the human condition: good vs. evil, human suffering and the meaning of life and death. To bring meaning to life and to deal with these various aspects of the human condition, rituals, ceremonies and the sacred myths of the gods and heroes were created. According to Carl Jung, myth is an essential part of the human psyche, which needs meaning and order in a world that is often chaotic.

Thus, the mythical structure centres round the myths we create and knowing what our heart wants us to know. Its clinical potency lies in understanding that myths are the stories our patients tell us and the stories we tell ourselves as to who we are. We can create a healing experience when we encourage our patients to positively reweave their stories and narrate from their Heart space as well as through the messages of their dreams and associated work with archetypes. Correspondingly, as practitioners, when we listen deeply from our Heart space to what is happening inside ourselves and our patients, we are connecting on a Heart-to-Heart or Shen-to-Shen basis. To achieve this heart attunement, the practitioner must first engage in self-cultivation, a life-long endeavour pursued via different practices such as Meditation with Breathwork, Inner Sensing or Qi Gong, which activate the energies of the mythical structure. Similarly, when we invoke the myths and the spirits of the acupuncture points in treating patients, or when we stay and hold the space in the discomfort of conflicting views or in a challenging situation of not knowing, we are entering into a mythical experience with our patients. This constant interplay is like dancing in rhythm with oneself and with the patient.

Integral structure: integration of all structures

When the archaic, magical, mythical and mental structures come together to form a dynamically harmonized structure, we have arrived at the integral whole that encompasses a multidimensional worldview. Such an orientation includes the different views expressed by human beings, considering what the environment (trees, plants, mountains) and animals might want. Clinically, the integral structure shows up when we take the time to reflect and to know when it is appropriate to act; when we have the 'Aha' moments (as when I discovered the golden key when working with my first exemplar patient); or engaging the lower dantian in Meditation.

The integral structure leads us to ask profoundly difficult and meaningful existential questions such as 'Who am I?', 'Where do I come from?', 'What is my past?', 'Where am I going?', 'What is my future?', 'How can I be free from the fear of death?' The transformation of the fear of death by living the life one is meant to live is, in Lorie Eve Dechar's words, the very essence of the alchemy of inner work. This work has profound societal and clinical implications, and this view gives us a wider definition of health and illness and thus shapes how healthcare services are made available and delivered.

This concludes a brief sketch of the clinical significance of Gebser's theory of consciousness that has so deeply influenced the understanding of my work and worldview. What follows next are some descriptions of the key Alchemical Healing tools I use with reference to the two patients presented earlier in this chapter.

INNER SENSING: A MAGICAL STRUCTURE EXPERIENCE

Inner Sensing was 'discovered' by Eugene Gendlin, an American philosopher and therapist, who named this phenomenon and developed a technique for incorporating it into a therapeutic process, which he called 'Focusing' (Cornell 1996). He realized that when clients only had an intellectual understanding of their problems, they did not achieve lasting positive resolution. Fundamental to lasting positive change was the client's ability to connect and describe their internal bodily sensations, which he called the 'felt sense'. Lorie Eve Dechar incorporated Focusing with Taoist inner alchemical practices to create a body-based practice she calls 'Inner Sensing', which she introduced to practitioners of Chinese medicine and their patients. Inner Sensing is a process whereby we access our inner knowing and tune in to our inner voice (tapping into the magical consciousness structure). This deep inner knowing is also experienced as a 'gut feeling', a bodily message that knows more than our mind knows. Thus, this bodily knowing bypasses the ever-dominant mental consciousness structure.

You can see how invaluable Inner Sensing was for the two patients described in this chapter as well as for myself as a practitioner. It provided me with a space and reference point to engage fully, be present, and to listen deeply to myself and to my patients. It is ultimately a healing process for the practitioner and patient. In sum, Inner Sensing is a body–mind alchemical practice used to get in touch with the authentic self. If you have never engaged in Inner Sensing before, I recommend working with a professional first. You can, however, make a start with the steps below.[14]

Before you do an Inner Sensing exercise:

1. Make sure that you are comfortable. Find a place where you cannot be disturbed. Sit comfortably with your feet touching the floor and your back well supported. Take a few slow breaths – inhaling and exhaling.

2. Put one hand where your heart area is and the other on your

lower dantian or belly. Bring your breath and your awareness to the areas where your hands are placed.

3. Keep breathing in and out slowly.

4. When ready, bring your awareness to your core, the area between your throat and the bottom of your pelvis.

5. Now ask yourself:

   a. What does my body know?

   b. What does my body feel?

   c. What does my body want me to know?

   d. What does my body need?

6. Take as much time as you need to listen and feel into your body.

7. You may feel a bodily sensation (felt sense) or receive a message from your body.

8. Without needing to change anything, imagine your bodily sensation as a friend sitting next to you. Feel her presence and connect with her.

9. Continue to breathe and listen to what your bodily sensation is telling you.

10. When you are ready, you can slowly come out of this exercise.

It is also a good idea to write down your experience after each Inner Sensing exercise.

DOING BY NOT DOING (WU WEI)

Learning to stay with the discomfort and the ability to do nothing until it is appropriate to act is a very important alchemical practice, which is useful for both the practitioner and the patient. In my clinical practice, there have been many such instances when all I could do was to be present and hold the space. Doing by not doing, or Wu Wei, comes from the Taoist principle of action in non-action, or the idea of going with the flow. It could also be interpreted as something that you have practised so hard and long that it has become effortless. When that happens, this is when mythical structure manifests.

THE SHEN

You may recall that the Shen is likened by the Taoists to a small bird, which is the spirit bird of the Heart and resides in its empty space. The Shen forms the very basis of the self and the soul. It is the light that shines within us, which gives us our special characteristics that make us uniquely who we are. When everything is in synchrony and balanced, the Shen lives harmoniously in our Heart space. However, emotional or spiritual turmoil can cause this light to dim and the bird to flee its nest. This metaphor of the small bird and its departure from the heart represents the loss of the soul or self as exemplified in my first patient who experienced anxiety, a disturbed sleep pattern, depression and a sense that something was not right. These symptoms are commonly reflected in many of my patients. When we practise a simple breath-in and breath-out with imagery of the small bird, we are simultaneously tapping into the healing energies of archaic and magical consciousness.

INTENTION AND THE POWER AND MYSTERY OF ACUPUNCTURE POINT NAMES

An acupuncture point is just an acupuncture point until you understand and work with its unique nature and function. When points are used with intention, they create a pathway to healing and transformation that communicates a clear signal to the body. This connection is the power of the magical structure.

The chosen points must be consistent with the patient's narrative. For example, PC 6 Nei Guan (Inner Gate) in patient no. 1 reflected that the Inner Gate had been shut for too long, that is, the secret she kept for so long. I felt that PC 6 provided an entry point that gently opened the Inner Gate to allow access to her healing energy to calm her restless Heart (Shen) and agitated mind so that she could be reconnected to the authentic self. This point supported inner clarity and connection to the Shen, and eventually the return of her joy and happiness.

Shame is guilt turned inwards, which, in turn, created many complex emotions such as anger, grief and depression. I suggested the use of ritual by burning incense to remember, honour and love herself as a grown-up and as a little girl as well as for her parents. This was because she had misgivings that her parents could not or would not protect her from the trauma she had suffered.

The power of naming things is also evident in the Internal Dragons treatment for patient no. 2. The idea of enlisting the help of a benevolent dragon is powerful to many of my patients. This image provided the catalyst that seemed to break down the barrier of patient no. 2's inability to access her emotions and opened the way for her 'Aha' moment...the manifestation of the power of the integral structure.

CONCLUDING THOUGHTS

In this chapter, we witnessed two patients who underwent the Alchemical Healing process. This begins with some kind of overwhelming challenge or symptom, often connected to a psychological and emotional issue, working through and staying with the pain and discomfort to eventually emerge having experienced some level of transformation. I have also highlighted the different Alchemical Healing tools and skills that were used, many of which do not require an acupuncture needle, to tap into the healing energies of the different structures of consciousness. I also gave an overview of the clinical significance of Gebser's theory of consciousness, and its ability to expand our worldview and provide a framework to understand the alchemical work.

Over the years, I have used many of the Alchemical Healing tools and skills in my clinical practice to great effect. However, the work of healing of psycho-emotional pain or distress is not for everyone. Its prerequisite is the patient's acknowledgement that work is called for and their willingness to stay engaged over time and in an ongoing relationship with the practitioner. The possibility of transformation conjures the visual image of the lotus stem's struggle to rise from the bottom of the muddy brown sludge of the pond to unfold above the water into a flawless lotus flower.

FURTHER READING

Holman, C.T. (2020) *Shamanism in Chinese Medicine.* London and Philadelphia, PA: Singing Dragon.

Jarrett, S.L. (2004) *Nourishing Destiny: The Inner Tradition of Chinese Medicine.* Stockbridge, MA: Spirit Path Press.

— CHAPTER 8 —

NURTURING AND NOURISHING OURSELVES: CHINESE MEDICINE APPROACH TO FOOD

INTRODUCTION

Nutrition is fundamental to our health. Yet confusion abounds as to what and what not to eat, not only for women with chronic pelvic pain, but also among those who do not suffer from chronic pain. This chapter does not aim to simplify a modern dietary approach; rather, it focuses on food from the Chinese medicine perspective. This is a complex and vast topic that requires an entire book to be written to do the subject justice. Therefore, I direct readers who are interested in deepening their knowledge to these two excellent books: *Chinese Natural Cures: Traditional Methods for Remedy and Prevention* by Henry C. Lu (Black Dog & Leventhal, 1999) and *Healing with Whole Foods: Asian Traditions and Modern Nutrition* by Paul Pitchford (North Atlantic Books, 2002).

My initial understanding of the Chinese medicine dietary approach is much influenced by my mother's cooking. I was nourished and nurtured in her household with delicious and traditional Chinese cooking that emphasized the balance of Yin–Yang and the five flavours (sour, bitter, sweet, spicy and salty). On hot and humid days, my mother cooked cooling herbal soups to counteract the heat and humidity.

Her mouth-watering chicken dish, which was cooked, with almost a pound of fresh root ginger and rice wine, especially for my sister who had just given birth, was memorable. This warming and nourishing dish supports the constitution of a woman after pregnancy and giving birth. I recall that almost everything we ate was cooked – stir-fried, steamed or poached – changing the energetics of food, which was unknown to me then. Thus, very early in my life, I absorbed my mother's wisdom on balancing foods that she had learned from her mother and grandmother. It was only years later that I realized that she was using food as medicine to optimize wellbeing and to minimize illness, which I thought was remarkable. This formative knowledge was broadened when I started my training in Chinese medicine and was further consolidated when I enrolled on a weekend course on the Chinese medicine dietary approach with Dr Jeffrey Yuen.[15]

FOOD AND THE DIGESTIVE SYSTEM: TWO KEY COMPONENTS

The Chinese medicine dietary approach emphasizes two key components: how we eat what we eat, and the health of the digestive system. The inclusion of these key components is noteworthy because most discussions on modern nutrition tend to focus on what food to eat or avoid, to the exclusion of the integrity of the digestive system. Chinese medicine considers the types of food we eat as well as the importance of the environment in which we consume them and the impact on the digestive system. Thus, if the digestive system is compromised, food that is difficult to digest will further burden the system, setting up a vicious cycle. Additionally, Chinese medicine understands that the balance of the different flavours (the five flavours) and energetics (Yin–Yang, cold, warm, hot) in food can affect our health via the five organs, namely the Liver, Heart, Spleen, Lungs and Kidneys. The digestive system is conceived in radically different ways from that of Western medicine. In Chinese medicine, the digestive organs consist of the Spleen[16] and Stomach.

In the clinical practice of Chinese medicine, the tongue is examined and used as one of the reliable guides to the overall status of the Spleen and Stomach, and the most appropriate foods to consume.

THE FIVE ELEMENTS, FLAVOURS AND COLOURS

Chinese medicine considers the unique flavours and energetics of meat, vegetables, fruits or seafood. These flavours are sour, bitter, sweet/bland, spicy and salty, which are associated with the Five Elements – Wood, Fire, Earth, Metal and Water, respectively (see Table 8.1). The Five Elements is a metaphor for describing the Qi (energy) in each season, food, all living beings and the universe. The sour flavour and the colour green are associated with Wood and the Liver, the bitter flavour and the colour red with Fire and the Heart, the sweet/bland flavour and the colour yellow with Earth and the Spleen and Stomach (the digestive organs), the spicy flavour and the colour white with Metal and the Lungs, and the salty flavour and the colour black with Water and the Kidneys. By including these five flavours in your diet, you are, in fact, balancing these five organs.

Flavours are important because they directly affect our internal organs, and thus our health. Flavours can be cooling, warming, hot or neutral. When a flavour is cooling or cold, it constricts and descends, and when it is hot, its movement tends to rise. Too much or not enough of one flavour can create disharmony. For example, too much sour-tasting food can hurt the Liver and Gall Bladder by creating stagnation. The key is to balance these flavours so as not to overburden or underserve any organ.

Table 8.1. The Five Elements and the related organ, flavour and colour

Element	Yin organ	Yang organ	Flavour	Colour
Wood	Liver	Gall Bladder	Sour	Green
Fire	Heart	Small Intestine	Bitter	Red
Earth	Spleen	Stomach	Sweet/bland	Yellow

Element	Yin organ	Yang organ	Flavour	Colour
Metal	Lungs	Large Intestine	Spicy	White
Water	Kidneys	Bladder	Salty	Black

The colour associated with each element is useful because it serves as a general guide as to what to include in our diet. For example, if you wish to nourish the Earth element, foods that are yellow in colour would be a good choice as yellow is associated with the Earth element. Similarly, foods that are black (such as black beans and black sesame seeds) nourish the Water element.

Wood: sour and green

Green-coloured and sour flavour benefit the Liver and Gall Bladder and are associated with the Wood element and Spring. Sour flavour tends to be Yin, cooling, and thus contracting and astringent. Sour flavour can be used in situations where there is profuse sweating, heavy menstrual flow, and bedwetting in children. Sour flavour assists the Liver in relaxing tight muscles. However, overindulgence in sour flavour can impede the digestion process, resulting in dryness. Too much sour food is harmful to the teeth.

Sour flavour mostly comes from citrus fruits, unripe fruits (mango or oranges) and vinegar. Besides the colour and flavour, the growth signature of vegetables (appearance) is useful as a guide to the type of energy they possess. Vegetables or plants that benefit the Liver and Gall Bladder are those that sprout such as alfalfa sprouts, and that grow straight and point upwards such as the stalks of vegetables and asparagus. These vegetables are said to contain Wood energy. Pulses or legumes such as peas and lentils are also packed with Wood energy. Vegetables can belong to several elements. For example, fennel can be classified as having Wood energy and some Earth energy because it is rounded, packed in and dense.

Fire: bitter and red

Bitter food affects the Heart and Small Intestines and is associated with Summer, the colour red and the Fire element. Bitter flavour tends to be Yin, cooling, drying, descending (promoting urination) and cleansing. Eaten in the appropriate amount, bitter flavour can help the digestive process, that is, the Stomach Qi, to descend. The drying property of a bitter cool flavour can help to dry Dampness. Too much bitter flavour in the diet can also result in dryness. Bitter-flavoured food can be used to clear Heart heat, which manifests as restlessness, insomnia and anxiety, accompanied by a red tongue with a red tip of the tongue. Sometimes there are tongue ulcers. Beans such as pinto beans and peas such as black eyed peas benefit the Heart, and it is a good idea to use them in soups with root vegetables, especially in the Summer, when or if it is hot and damp.

Slightly bitter-flavoured food comes from vegetables such as snow peas, spinach, bitter greens such as kale, collard greens, Chinese broccoli, mustard greens and celery. Coffee and tea are considered to have a bitter flavour.

Sunflower seeds absorb a significant amount of solar energy, and food that is red in colour, for example strawberries, red beans, tomatoes, apples and watermelon, generally benefits the Heart and Small Intestines.

Bitter food, as opposed to slightly bitter-flavoured food, is not very tasty and thus not used too much in the culinary world, except, of course, dark chocolate, as long as it has a high percentage of cacao (such as 70 per cent). Chocolate also goes to the digestive organs, the Spleen and Stomach, because it is sweet. Thus, taken in appropriate amounts, chocolate can be good for health.

Earth: sweet/bland and yellow

Sweet flavour affects the Spleen and Stomach and is associated with the Earth element, late Summer and the colour yellow. Sweet flavour has a tonifying effect: it can tonify Yin or Yang. Sweet and warm flavours help to build Qi, Yang, Yin and Blood. Sweet and cool flavours are usually moistening. A sweet flavour can also help the Spleen to transform and transport, that is, it is good for the digestive process. In appropriate amounts, a sweet flavour is stimulating and promotes digestion and relaxes spasms in smooth muscles. Hence a little dessert (not too rich), such as a small piece of dark chocolate to end a meal, helps with digestion. However, a meal that has an overabundance of sweet flavours can create Dampness and Phlegm, which, in Chinese medicine, is an accumulation of pathological fluid that impedes the healthy functioning of the body. When Dampness invades the Lungs, it manifests as Phlegm, especially after eating food that is difficult to digest such as milk (especially if you are lactose intolerant) or greasy food. Symptoms related to Phlegm are coughing, a sore throat and coughing up mucus, for example.

Sweet flavour comes mostly from carbohydrates such as grains and root vegetables. Grains are associated with the Earth element and when chewed for long enough, there is a slightly sweet taste. Grains can be drying or moistening and can break up stagnation. Examples of drying grains are wheat, rye, quinoa and buckwheat. These are more suitable for a weak digestive system with poor transformation and transportation (e.g., Spleen Qi deficiency), and stagnation of the Spleen and Stomach Qi.

Examples of moistening grains are oats, barley, millet and corn grits, and these are more suitable for the Stomach as it likes wetness. Millet is the most moistening of these grains, and when roasted it drains Dampness and helps with morning sickness in pregnancy. Corn grits nourish Yin (moisture), and thus are useful for dryness. Moistening grains are helpful for Stomach Fire, which manifests as acid reflux, dyspepsia, ulcers and an insatiable appetite. The tongue coating is yellow and thick. There is usually a crack (either horizontal or vertical) in the centre of the tongue and the tongue body is red and dry.

White rice that is polished is more suitable for people with a weak or compromised digestive system. Brown rice, which is more difficult to digest, is thus for people with a more robust digestive system.

Besides grains, other foods that are associated with the Earth element and sweet flavour are yams, sweet potatoes and carrots, all of which are excellent in soups or as part of a main meal. Foods that are yellow in colour and rounded are generally associated with the Earth element, as are root vegetables. Pumpkin and watermelon seeds and chickpeas are good for the Spleen and Stomach. These grains and vegetables also provide bulk for the digestive system and thus help to prevent constipation.

Overconsumption of sweet flavours that come from highly refined sugars such as table sugar, soft drinks and cakes may make endometriosis-associated pain worse. This is because endometriosis is an inflammatory condition that can be fuelled by too much sugar in the diet.

Metal: spicy and white

Spicy foods affect the Lung and Large Intestine and are associated with Autumn, the Metal element and the colour white. Spicy flavour is dispersing and directs Qi upwards, and is therefore Yang in nature. Spicy flavour stimulates the taste buds, opens pores (encourages sweating), moves stagnation by promoting the circulation of Qi and Blood and has an uplifting effect, and can thus be helpful if someone is feeling a little down. Too much spicy food can injure the digestive system.

Spicy flavour can come from seeds (cinnamon, coriander leaf or seeds, anise seeds, turmeric and cumin seeds), roots (ginger root) and nuts (cardamom, nutmeg). These seeds are warming and are helpful for people with a weak digestion. I often make a warming chai tea, with cinnamon, ginger root, cardamom and anise seeds, during the Winter months.

Spicy flavour can be acrid and pungent. Acrid flavour is minty and refreshing. Examples of acrid food are basil, spearmint, mint, lemongrass, parsley and rosemary. Acrid food such as mint is warming, and thus its energy moves up and out. Examples of pungent food are onions, garlic, leeks, spring onions (scallions), shallots, chives and ginger. A small amount of pungent food helps to open the sinuses and promote appetite.

Water: salty and black

Salty flavour benefits the Kidneys and Urinary Bladder and is associated with Water element, Winter and the colour black. Salty-flavoured food is cooling, moistening and descending, and tends to go inward as well as having a softening effect on hardness or lumps. Examples of salty-flavoured food that is cooling (reduces inflammation), and softening are seaweed and salt. Seaweed can be used in soups or salads, and can be really delicious. Sometimes I eat it toasted. However, a diet that has too much salty flavour can interfere with fluid metabolism, and make Dampness worse.

Salty-flavoured foods come from molluscs (clams, oysters, conch, mussels, scallops, snails and abalone) and provide protein in our diet. Snails can help to reduce the severity of a urinary tract infection as they go to the Bladder. Conch is helpful in cases of frequent urination, but has to be cooked for a long time, otherwise it is chewy and difficult to digest.

If molluscs or other seafood are not allowed or tolerated in your diet, you can always use seeds because all seeds benefit the Kidneys, especially those that are black in colour such as black sesame seeds. Raw seeds are Yin but toasting or roasting them makes them more Yang. I recall from my childhood a dessert where raw black sesame seeds with honey were cooked to a thick consistency to replenish the essence of the Kidneys. We were only allowed a small bowl each because consuming too much could be too sticky and Damp-inducing. Toasted black sesame seeds that are sprinkled over cucumbers are not only delicious; they are also indicated in cases of incomplete voiding of urine. In Chinese medicine, essence is a vital substance that you inherit from your parents, and it provides the foundation for reproduction, growth and health.

Another seed that brings energy to the Kidney and the Heart is the sunflower seed. I find that one of the best ways to consume sunflower seeds is to toast them and sprinkle them over salad and morning breakfast cereals. Toasting sunflower seeds makes them more Yang (warming), which counterbalances the Yin of the salad. Other food that is good for the Kidneys is kidney beans, black beans and other dark-coloured beans.

If you are feeling that your body needs cooling, try some dandelion greens. These are considered salty and cooling, and thus an excellent anti-inflammatory. Gently steam them and then toss them in balsamic vinegar and olive oil. Just before you eat them, sprinkle over some of your favourite untoasted seeds or nuts.

THE YIN–YANG OF FOOD
The spectrum of Yin–Yang

Human nature as well as food can also be understood as more Yin or more Yang or simply a gradation of Yin and Yang. Food such as fowl (chicken, duck) is considered most Yang and warming (left on the spectrum) and food such as fruits (all types of melon) is said to be most Yin (right on the spectrum) (see Table 8.2). What we are referring to is the 'energetics of food'.

Table 8.2. Yin–Yang food spectrum

Most Yang (warming)	Fowl	Mammals	Amphibians	Shellfish	Seeds Legumes Nuts Grains Vegetables	[AQ] Fruits (Lungs)	Most Yin (cooling)

The concept of Yin–Yang underpins Chinese medicine (Zhong Yi), which is translated as the 'medicine of the centre or middle'. Clinically, this is done by balancing Yin and Yang to bring the patient back to the centre, using approaches such as acupuncture, modification in the diet or lifestyle, as well as the way we handle our emotions.

Yin–Yang is a spectrum and used as a comparison of two entities. It means that Yin is not completely dark or lacking in energy and Yang is not total brightness. Rather, Yin–Yang is relative and always at work to balance itself. In Chinese medicine, Yin can be understood as less bright (less Qi (energy)) when compared with Yang (most Qi (energy)). Yin can be described as a cloudy day where the sunlight is filtered through the cloud, and Yang is a sunny day where there is direct sunlight (like around 12 pm in the tropics). Energetically speaking, Yin–Yang can be understood as our life force circulating at different stages of the day and in our lives. The life force is felt as degrees of warmth, without which it will be totally cold and dark, as in death.

Yin is watery and is considered cooling; Yang is more dense, compact and warming. If you are on the cooler side (Yin), you may want to consume foods that are warming (Yang). Likewise, if you always feel hot (Yang), you may wish to have cooler foods (Yin). Thus, consuming a mix of Yin and Yang foods, those based on the season and your individual constitution will help bring you to the middle, that is, balance.

Cooking vs. raw

It is generally believed that raw food contains higher levels of nutrients than cooked food, and is therefore better for health and wellbeing. Recall that the Chinese medicine dietary approach takes into consideration the integrity of the digestive organs (Spleen and Stomach) as well as the food we consume. Cooking breaks down the food, and cooking food for a long time breaks down food even more. Cooking pre-digests the food, which aids the functions of the Spleen and Stomach. Hence, herbal and food tonics are cooked for a long time to render it easier for the digestive system to do its work. Congee (jook), which is rice that has been cooked for over an hour or two, is another excellent example of prolonged cooking to aid in the absorption of nutrients. It is therefore especially suitable for people with a weak digestive system. If the digestive system is weak, raw food will likely compromise the digestive system further, and its nutrients will not be absorbed. Thus, eating raw food might do more harm than good. However, a strong digestive system is more likely to be able to cope with raw food. Thus, it depends on the health of the digestive organs as to whether it is better to eat cooked or raw food.

In general, for women with chronic pelvic pain, it is a good idea to avoid eating too much raw food and icy cold drinks, especially if their

NURTURING AND NOURISHING OURSELVES

pain responds to warmth or is made worse by cold. Cold drinks and food tend to decrease circulation and make the pain worse.

Cooking not only breaks down food, but it also changes its nature. For example, roasting or deep-frying a chicken makes it more Yang (more warming), while poaching it makes it more Yin (less warming). Vegetables when eaten raw are more Yin (cooling) compared with steaming, stir-frying or deep-frying (warming) them. Soaking grains, legumes or seeds before cooking renders them more digestible, and thus less likely to produce bloating. A Yin fruit such as a banana can be transformed into a Yang fruit by deep-frying. Eggs are considered Yin but if you eat too much, they become Yang.

OPTIMIZING HEALTH: HOW FOOD IS CONSUMED

Chinese medicine recognizes the importance of not only the nature of food but also how it is consumed. Feeding yourself and/or your family with nutritious food is no guarantee that your body/their bodies will benefit from it because other factors can interfere with the integrity of the Spleen and Stomach. Here are some of the ways to maximize the functions of the Spleen and Stomach as well as the enjoyment of food.

Create a shopping list mindfully

Our body protects us and is the vehicle that feeds our mind and animates our spirit and soul. Thus, how and what we feed ourselves matters enormously. To avoid impulse buying, plan your meals and create a shopping list. Shopping and cooking mindfully are some of the best ways to show deep respect and love for ourselves and for our Earth. We can practise mindful shopping and eating to a point that they become a habit; however, we have to do it regularly and consistently, as permanent change doesn't happen overnight! Can you imagine if everyone acquired this habit how much better off we would be!

I believe there is a growing awareness that the Earth's resources are finite. I remember many years ago, before eating the leaves of beetroot became fashionable, the farmers in Union Square's market in New

York City kept the leaves and stalks for the locals who knew the secret of using these delicious parts that many did not know about. It makes me feel better now that supermarkets in the UK have started selling vegetables such as carrots or peppers that are perfectly imperfectly shaped (they do not conform to their idea of a perfect vegetable) at a lower price instead of binning them.

Create a calm emotional tone

We have all, at some point or another, experienced butterflies in our stomach or the urge to urinate frequently when we feel stressed or anxious. This is because the digestive system feels the effect of stress or anxiety as it is constantly 'talking' with the nervous system. When the Qi in the body is taken up by stress or anxiety, there is precious little for the Spleen and Stomach to do their work. It is therefore not a good idea to eat when you are in a state of high anxiety or stress. However, we can interrupt the 'conversation' between the digestive and the nervous systems, using the notion that intentional breathing is the language of the nervous system. Give yourself a few minutes and try any of the breathing techniques that I outline in Chapter 9. Once you feel calmer and less stressed, you can begin your meal, but not before.

A new patient reported that she could not get enough air into her lungs even if she inhaled deeply. Further, she felt that there was a 'lump' in her throat, especially during mealtimes. She was afraid she would choke on her food. Thus, she ate what she said was 'junk' food throughout the day, to avoid the choking sensation at mealtimes.

During our consult, I noticed she was rather hesitant in sharing her health information, and she looked ill at ease in her body. On further asking, she revealed that she was anxious and very stressed about her chronic pelvic pain and the situation at home. She used to do Flow Yoga but had stopped as she was worried that the Yoga might be aggravating her pelvic pain. I suggested some of the breathing techniques and Yin Yoga instead of Flow Yoga, which is more strenuous. Importantly, the key is to deeply and intentionally engage with the practice on a regular basis. She reported significant improvement, and that the breathing before mealtimes really helped her.

Create a calm environment

Before you eat, set and create an attractive dinner table so that you are tempted to sit at the table rather than in front of the television while eating. For example, a simple red rose in a small vase can create a very different feel to your table. Get rid of any distraction to the enjoyment of your meal, such as having the television or radio on or trying to read text messages or emails on your phone. Make a commitment to yourself to focus on your food, be conscious of your breath-in and breath-out, slow down, wake up and smell the roses/coffee.

Enjoy: food is a gift to all the senses

One of the most precious aspects of eating is enjoyment. The different flavours and textures of food not only should nourish and nurture our body, mind, spirit and soul, but are also a gift to all our senses: smell, sight, taste and hearing. Remember to enjoy the aroma that comes with the cooking of your food – a gift to your sense of smell/nose. Once the cooking is done, plate your food beautifully – a gift to your sense of aesthetics/eyes. Then savour the taste as you chew and listen to the crunching of the vegetables or nuts – a gift to your taste buds and ears. So spring alive and enjoy your food.

One bowl eating Meditation: enjoy in small bites and portions

There is a useful Zen Buddhist practice called the 'one bowl eating meditation' (Dechar 2006, p.228). This practice helps to prevent overeating by portion control and mindful eating. You are allowed to fill your one bowl, but you cannot go back for more. Enjoy your food mindfully by taking small bites, chewing slowly, noticing the essence and flavours to enhance the enjoyment of food as well as to encourage communication between the digestive and nervous systems. The result is that you leave the dinner table feeling satiated instead of feeling unsatisfied, which results in craving and snacking throughout the day. When on holiday in France, I was struck and impressed by the wait staff who invariably asked if we were satiated at the end of the meal, which was enjoyed over several hours. I believe we should take note of the deep reverence the French have for food, and thus it is important, perhaps sacrilegious even, not to enjoy your meal.

Undereating

The Spleen and Stomach do not function well with infrequent meals. They like it less when there is severe restriction of food intake due to dieting because of damage to the Qi and Yang of the Spleen and Stomach. It is better all round to eat small, nutritious meals.

Optimal mealtime

There is no such thing as a perfect diet or a perfect time to eat. Based on the Chinese energy clock, the best time to eat the biggest meal is between 7 am and 11 am, that is, breakfast, when the Stomach and Spleen Qi are most active. Lunch and dinner could then be a relatively light meal. However, whether we eat a big breakfast or big dinner depends on the individual. For example, if the Stomach and Spleen Qi are deficient, a big breakfast may not be appropriate. Rather, small and frequent meals would be more suitable. An elderly person with a weak Kidney may benefit from eating a bigger meal in the evening, as Kidney energy tends to be regenerated at night. If the Liver is weak, eating a late dinner may help build the Liver. Thus, the optimal time for meals depends on the individual's constitution and health status. However, the functions of the Spleen and Stomach are optimized when food is consumed on a regular basis. Therefore, evaluate what time is best for you by paying attention to your bodily reactions to each mealtime, and then establish a routine and stick to it.

A DIFFERENT WORLDVIEW OF THE DIGESTIVE SYSTEM: THE STOMACH AND SPLEEN ORGANS

If you are new to Chinese medicine, I invite you to temporarily let go of your Western medicine knowledge about the Spleen and Stomach so that it does not get in the way of seeing and understanding Chinese medicine's concepts. So, bundle up your Western knowledge into a parcel, and leave it outside the door.

Functions of the Spleen and Stomach

ROTTING AND RIPENING OF FOOD

An important function of Stomach Qi is to 'cook' the ingested food and fluids in preparation for the Spleen. The Stomach is often likened to a cooking pot. To cook the food and fluids we consume, the Stomach requires heat. Therefore, consumption of foods and fluids that are too cold or even too hot injure the functions of the Stomach.

TRANSFORMATION AND TRANSPORTATION OF FOOD ESSENCES

The Spleen transforms the prepared food and fluids into food essences and transports them to the Lungs and Heart, which is then turned into food essences (Qi and Blood). The food essences are also sent to the Small Intestine by the descending function of the Stomach Qi. If you often have nausea, regurgitation, hiccoughs, belching and a sensation of fullness after eating, it may indicate that your Stomach Qi is not functioning at its best.

In contrast, the Spleen Qi rises, and if it is weak or impaired, it will be unable to transport the food essences upwards to the Lungs and Heart. If you experience chronic Spleen Qi deficiency, you may find it difficult to focus and concentrate, and your thinking is muddled and foggy. There may also be prolapse of various internal organs such as the uterus, bladder or anus.

PRODUCING FLUIDS

The Stomach likes wetness and dislikes dryness, while the Spleen likes dryness and dislikes wetness. The Stomach requires fluids to break down the food just as a juicer requires fluids to extract the essence from fruits and vegetables. When there is a lack of fluids, the Stomach is unable to function optimally; thus there will be thirst and poor digestion. The Spleen sorts out the usable and unusable parts of the food essences and fluids.

KEEPING BLOOD IN THE VESSELS
A healthy Spleen keeps blood in the vessels. When the Spleen is deficient, bruising or bleeding may come easily.

CONTROLLING THE MUSCLES AND FOUR LIMBS
The Spleen's function is to transform and transport food essences to nourish the body; specifically it maintains the tone and strength of the muscles and the four limbs. Chronic digestive issues, such as type 2 diabetes, may result in poor muscle tone and weakness in the arms and legs.

Common problems in the Stomach and Spleen
This section highlights some of the common disharmonies of the Stomach and Spleen (although it is not a complete list).

STOMACH QI DEFICIENCY
When you have discomfort in the epigastrium, lack of appetite, loose stools, tiredness (especially in the morning) accompanied by a pale tongue (presence of Cold), you might have Stomach Qi deficiency. According to the Chinese energetic clock, the Stomach's peak activity is between 7 am and 9 am, which would explain why tiredness is experienced in the morning. You may recall that the Stomach Qi descends when it is functioning normally; however, when it is deficient, it fails to descend, creating a sense of discomfort in the epigastrium. When the Stomach is not working efficiently, it impacts on the Spleen, resulting in Spleen Qi deficiency. In both cases, the tongue colour is pale.

SPLEEN QI DEFICIENCY

Spleen Qi deficiency may come about due to Stomach Qi deficiency. Spleen Qi deficiency is common and underpins all Spleen disharmonies such as Spleen Qi sinking, Spleen not controlling Blood or Spleen Yang deficiency. Basically, in Spleen Qi deficiency the Spleen's transformation and transportation functions are impaired to varying degrees depending on the seriousness of the deficiency. The Spleen's inability to transform fluids leads to Dampness, a condition that the Spleen dislikes.

You can recognize Spleen Qi deficiency when there is no appetite, loose stools, tiredness and abdominal distension after eating. The most common causes of Spleen Qi deficiency are eating either too much or too little, overconsumption of cold and raw foods, eating irregularly or severely restricting food intake as well as chronic overthinking.

The colour of the tongue is pale or normal and the sides of the tongue may be scalloped.

STOMACH COLD

This condition is like Stomach Qi deficiency with added Cold (deficient), and is closely linked to Spleen Yang deficiency (described later). If you have cold limbs, loose stools, no thirst and a preference for warm drinks and foods as well as a pale tongue, you may have Stomach Cold.

Food to include

Think of a diet that strengthens the Spleen and Stomach. This would include appropriately cooked food such as grains (carbohydrates), small amounts of protein and lightly cooked vegetables.

Sweet or neutral food such as rice, quinoa, roasted barley, pumpkin, sweet potatoes and millet are sweet and thus have an affinity with the Stomach and Spleen. Root vegetables are also excellent for the Stomach and Spleen. It is a good idea to use small amounts of pungent flavours such as onions, leeks, garlic, fresh ginger and fennel.

It is important to cook your food well. Grains require a longer cooking time. In general, the more food is cooked (be it meat or rice), the less taxing it is for the Stomach and Spleen. Congee (jook) is a very good example of rice that has undergone prolonged cooking and is thus ideal for people dealing with a chronic illness or convalescing. There are many recipes in the excellent book, *The Book of Jook: A Healthy Alternative to the Typical Western Breakfast*, by Bob Flaws (Blue Poppy Press, Inc., 1995). Green leafy vegetables do not require prolonged cooking; rather, gentle steaming or stir-frying to a crisp makes the food more appealing, digestible and nutritious.

Food to exclude or avoid

Exclude or avoid Damp-generating food such as ice cream, sugar, chocolate and pastries, and cold-natured food such as salad, raw vegetables and fruit juices.

Do not skip meals or eat while working or driving.

SPLEEN YANG DEFICIENCY

This disharmony evolves in the same way as Spleen Qi deficiency. Spleen Yang deficiency shows up as someone who has no appetite, abdominal distension after eating, feels cold and tired, has cold limbs, loose stools and sometimes oedema. Spleen Yang can be likened to the fire that is doing the cooking and heating. Thus, when there is Spleen Yang deficiency, it is as if the fire has been turned off, which disables the transformation and transportation functions of the Spleen. As a result, the limbs are cold and oedema is present, as well as a wet, puffy and pale tongue.

Food to include

The food to include is similar to that recommended for Qi Deficiency. In addition, it is a good idea to include warmer foods such as parsnips, lamb, beef, chicken, stewed fruits (dark-coloured fruits such as apricots and plums), dry ginger (instead of fresh ginger), cloves, cinnamon and star anise.

Food to exclude or avoid
Avoid all manner of raw food and iced drinks.

STOMACH HEAT/FIRE

This is caused by overconsuming hot spicy foods, meat, alcohol and coffee, and smoking. If this condition is not rectified, the Heat will consume the Stomach fluids (Stomach Yin) leading to Stomach Yin deficiency. Stomach Heat can escalate into Stomach Fire (a more severe form of Stomach Heat), where the pain in the Stomach region is more severe and burning. In this case, the hunger is constant. Other symptoms include sour regurgitation, nausea, severe thirst with a desire for cold drinks, constipation, swelling and bleeding gums as well as bad breath and a thick yellow tongue coating.

Food to include
Because of the excess Heat, it is important to clear the Heat by eating lightly cooked foods and raw fruits and vegetables that are cooling. Specific foods that are good for reducing the Heat in the Stomach are grains such as rice, barley, oats and millet; vegetables such as celery, spinach, cucumber, lettuce, radishes (daikon), avocado, watercress and broccoli; and fruits such as apples, pears and watermelon; as well as mung beans, yoghurt, oysters and clams.

Food to exclude or reduce
It is a good idea to reduce the intake of meat, alcohol, spicy food (wasabi, chillies, mustard, curries) and coffee.

Do not smoke.

STOMACH YIN DEFICIENCY

The key word here is dryness – a dry mouth and throat, dry stools and thirst, with no desire to drink. Additionally, there is no appetite and a subjective feeling of Heat in the afternoon. The tongue is red, has no coating and a peeled (patchy) centre, where the Stomach and Spleen are reflected. Stomach Yin deficiency is commonly caused by chronic irregular eating patterns.

Food to include

Because there is a significant amount of dryness, food that is moisturizing is recommended. A diet that has a combination of green leafy vegetables, root vegetables, grains such as wheat, as well as seeds and beans and a small amount of animal protein is desirable. Root vegetables, beans and meat can be made into stews and soups to improve fluid and moisture levels to nourish the Stomach Yin. Other foods to nourish the Stomach Yin are barley, millet, tofu, banana, plums, mung beans, sweet potatoes and asparagus.

Food to exclude or reduce

See the list in 'Stomach Heat/Fire'.

CONCLUDING THOUGHTS

Nutrition in Chinese medicine includes not only the food we eat and how we eat, but also our digestive system. Foods have different flavours and colours and are associated with the seasons and the organs. Blending the different flavours and colours ensures a balanced diet, which is fundamental to health and one of the best ways to nourish and nurture ourselves. In deciding what to eat, Chinese medicine also considers the health status or constitution of the individual. The conditions under which we eat our food have an impact on the digestive system, and thus how food is digested. In summary, Chinese medicine nutrition is a comprehensive approach to health and wellness, and one of the many ways to nourish and nurture ourselves.

FURTHER READING

Lu, H.C. (2005) *Chinese Natural Cures: Traditional Methods for Remedy and Prevention.* New York: Black Dog & Leventhal Publishers, Inc.

Maciocia, G. (1989) *The Foundations of Chinese Medicine.* London: Churchill Livingstone.

Maclean, W. and Lyttleton, J. (2002) *Clinical Handbook of Internal Medicine, Vol. 2.* Sydney: University of Western Sydney.

Pitchford, P. (2002) *Healing with Whole Foods: Asian Traditions and Modern Nutrition* (3rd edn). Berkeley, CA: North Atlantic Books.

Yuen, J. (2007) Lecture notes on 'Chinese dietary approach'. 11 and 12 August.

—— CHAPTER 9 ——

CREATING A TOOLBOX TO NURTURE AND NOURISH OURSELVES

YANG SHENG: NURTURING, NOURISHING AND PROTECTING OURSELVES

In writing this chapter, I have borrowed the important concept of Yang Sheng from ancient Chinese medicine. 'Yang' means to nourish and nurture, and 'Sheng' means life, birth and vitality. Thus, Yang Sheng involves tending to aspects of ourselves that need nourishing, nurturing, healing and protecting as well as aspects that are flourishing. To practise Yang Sheng, we make use of the potency of our innate healing power to heal and take care of our physical body, emotions, feelings and thoughts, and the realms of the spirits. I have woven into this chapter the different sources of our innate healing energies and how to access them through practices such as Meditation, visualization, Yoga or Qi Gong that have Breathwork as a common thread. I have also used concepts such as the Five Spirits from the Five Elements theory and Jean Gebser's theory of consciousness, discussed in Chapter 7. To recap, in the Five Elements theory, this healing energy resides in the five spirits (Shen), which has parallels with Gebser's theory of consciousness. The five spirits are the Hun, Shen, Yi, Po and Zhi, which are associated with the Liver, Heart, Earth, Metal and Water, respectively.

INTENTION AND THE YI SPIRIT

In any healing practice, it is important to recruit the power of our intention that resides with the Yi spirit of the Earth element. It helps us to create our intention and focus our attention. For example, the Yi spirit can direct and focus the Qi (intention and attention) to a particular area of the body that needs healing or love by creating a pathway and signal for the Qi and Blood to follow accordingly. This unique and beneficial interaction among these entities is very important, and it is thus often used in the clinical practice of Chinese medicine. In short, Qi follows where the mind goes and what the mind focuses on. An intention might be as simple as to breathe in peace of mind and to breathe out something that no longer serves us that we need to let go of. This intentional Breathwork is a form of active Meditation and is manifested by the Yi, the Earth spirit. Focusing our attention on an intention is a skill that requires cultivation and patience; you can practise this daily and in small steps. It is a major aspect of the meditative practice of Chinese martial arts such as Kung Fu and Qi Gong, as well as acupuncture, and can be applied to Meditation, Breathwork and Yoga.

VISUALIZATION

Visualization is as important as bringing an intention to your practice, and they work together. Visualization is about imagining and creating specific images and directing them to a particular purpose, such as to address symptoms of a disease, reduce pain, relax and enhance a sense of wellbeing. During Breathwork you can incorporate a visualization routine such as an image of a healthy self or a colour that has a meaning for you (visual imagery), listening to your favourite piece of music (auditory), eating a delicious piece of fruit (gustatory) or smelling your favourite scent (olfactory). Just to practise, imagine yourself in the kitchen squeezing a lemon. You can visualize the smell of the lemon and the sharp, sour taste of its juice, and these should make your mouth water. Once you've got the idea, try 'Invitation to Return Home' presented later in this chapter.

First let's begin with a slow Breathwork practice.

SLOW BREATHWORK, ANYTIME, ANYWHERE

When we engage in this slow Breathwork, we are tapping into the revitalizing and healing energies of the Zhi spirit of the Kidney and the archaic consciousness in Gebser's structure of consciousness (see Chapter 7). If you have never engaged in any conscious Breathwork, here are some tips to get started. As in all Breathwork, it is important to do your breath-in and breath-out slowly. If it is done too quickly, you may feel slightly dizzy. If that is the case, stop and wait awhile, and then restart at a slower pace.

You don't need any special equipment, just the following:

1. Set an intention for this practice.

2. Sit down comfortably, come into yourself, and focus your attention on each normal and even breath-in and breath-out.

3. Place one hand over your heart area and one hand over your belly button area, which is the dantian (where the original Source Qi (energy) of the Water element and the archaic consciousness is situated); when in a public area, cross your arms over the diaphragm area, just below the breasts.

4. Your mind will wander to all sorts of different things, places or 'to do' lists. Say 'hello' to these wandering thoughts and then say 'goodbye'.

5. Continue to take a slow breath-in and breath-out into where your hands are.

6. Imagine breathing down into the dantian and enter into the area of your healing energy.

7. Notice any slight changes in your body or mind.

8. Practise once daily for a few minutes for several weeks.

With practice you will notice that you feel calmer and more centred. When this happens, you know that you are using the healing energies of your Water element, the archaic consciousness. When you are ready, you can embark on something more involved. Or you can just stay here and enjoy the benefits of this simple practice. Importantly, it is free, and you can do it anywhere, anytime, yes, even in public, for example while waiting to see your doctor, having dental work or when you are on the bus and if you start to feel anxious. This simple and easy-to-use Breathwork can be used as the basis of any mind–body practice.

It is also a good idea to keep a journal to chart your progress.

BREATHWORK AND VISUALIZATION FOR ANXIOUS DAYS: 'INVITATION TO RETURN HOME'

This powerful heart-centred practice combines Breathwork and visualization and enlists the healing energies of the Shen spirit of the Heart, which could be said to be Gebser's mythical consciousness. It is excellent for anxiety and restlessness, and for times when you feel that you are not quite yourself. These symptoms reflect the agitation of the Shen. In ancient Chinese medicine the symbol for the Shen is a delicate white or red bird that resides in the empty space of the Heart. When there is emotional and spiritual agitation, this bird is unable to return home to the Heart space. This practice warmly invites the bird to return home safely.

Begin with the 'Slow Breathwork, anytime, anywhere' routine. Then visualize a white or red bird that represents the Shen spirit of the Heart. Once you have got the image, gently invite this bird to return home to the Heart space. Take your time to do this:

1. Adopt a friendly and welcoming attitude towards yourself and the little bird.

2. Make sure you have one hand over the heart and the other over the belly button area.

3. Continue to take a slow breath-in and breath-out. Always return to your breath if you catch your mind wandering off to someplace else.

4. When you are ready, gently invite the bird to return home to your Heart space.

5. Imagine the bird settling comfortably into the Heart space.

6. Imagine the light of your Shen shining on the bird.

7. Then observe without judgement your bodily sensation.

8. You will begin to regain a sense of calmness and warmth in the Heart area.

9. Continue to breathe in and breathe out until you are ready to stop.

10. Thank yourself and the bird.

THE POWER OF NEGATIVE SELF-TALK

Yesterday I was clever, so I wanted to change the world,
Today I am wise, so I am changing myself. (Rumi)

Almost everyone engages in negative self-talk at one time or another. Negative self-talk is very powerful, and yet we do it to ourselves all the time. We tell ourselves stories of how we are not good enough, not intelligent enough, not slim enough or not beautiful enough. In short, we simply believe that we are not enough. This kind of negative self-talk has the power to diminish us, stops us from believing in ourselves, limits our potential and makes us unhappy. This is because we start to believe the negative narratives we weave for ourselves. Sooner or later, they become our reality. Just as negative narratives have the power to trap us in an adverse manner, positive narratives have the power to free us to move forward in a beneficial manner. So let's be wise and change our narratives to ones that will serve us well.

As an example, I would like to share how I transform my negative 'reality', which I had mistaken to be the truth, into a positive meaningful one. This is another instance of accessing the power of the mythical or the Shen consciousness to guide us to the right action.

Changing our narrative and ourselves: connecting with the mythical (Shen) consciousness

This is the story I have been telling myself for the longest time, and I am *not* sticking to it any more. I used to die a little when people asked if my name had a meaning. I would try to dodge and be evasive. Why? Because my name, 'Ooi Thye', directly translates as 'love brother'. My parents gave me this name hoping that it would bring forth a son in the next pregnancy, because up to that point, they only had one son but three daughters. Instead, they got me, yet another daughter. I tell myself what a disappointment I must have been to my parents. I carried this story inside my head, believing that 'I am a disappointment, and my name is an embarrassment'. My parents would have been saddened to learn about this belief for surely I was never a disappointment, and my name was never an embarrassment.

I never shared this narrative that I created for myself with anyone until I realized what I was doing to myself. As part of my transformational journey, and with the help of my Alchemical Healer, I reframed my story into a comforting and powerful one, which gives me back *me*. It was a light bulb moment. My name, 'Ooi Thye', is my inner spirit brother, my inner strength and soul mate who puts me in touch with my inner archetype, which is infused with healing energies. I can and I do go to him for help, share my joy and success and many more things. In sum, we need to tell, feel and talk about ourselves in a radically different way in order to change our emotional and mind state to a positive one.

AFFIRMATIONS

In Chapter 6, I mentioned Wang Fengyi's approach to healing in which changing your life's narratives and affirmations through chanting are some of the tools for emotional and spiritual healing. These affirmations focused on being in touch with the virtues of the five archetypes of the Five Elements theory, but in my clinical practice I adapt his idea and co-create affirmations that are meaningful to each patient. Below are some affirmations that you can use when working with your patients, to help them get in touch with their inner archetypes or elements.

Begin with Breathwork
Every morning, before you get out of bed:

1. Take a slow, deep breath-in (count 1, 2, 3, 4, 5).

2. Take a slow, deep breath-out (1, 2, 3, 4, 5, 6).

3. Repeat steps (1) and (2).

Repeat your affirmations
Repeat one or several of the affirmations below X times either silently to yourself or aloud.

Affirmations to be in touch with your:

1. Wood archetype:

   I have a plan and direction.

   I have compassion for myself and others.

   I am accomplished.

   I start and complete tasks.

2. Fire archetype:

   I am deeply respectful.

I love myself and others.

I am connected with myself and others.

I am truthful.

I am happy.

3. Earth archetype:

I trust myself and others.

I am reliable.

I nurture and nourish myself and others.

I take responsibility for my mistakes and I do not blame others.

4. Metal archetype:

I do not judge myself and others harshly.

I am grateful.

I am logical and precise.

I contribute to the community selflessly.

5. Water archetype:

I am humble and wise.

I am creative.

I am soft and harmonious and I go with the flow.

I am not a victim.

The key is to do these affirmations with sincerity so that they touch your Heart and make a connection with the respective archetype. Remember to check in with your feelings and thoughts throughout the day. If you catch yourself going on a journey of negative self-talk, interrupt yourself as follows.

Interrupt your negative self-talk

1. *Stop.*

2. Take a slow, deep breath-in (count 1, 2, 3, 4, 5).

3. Take a slow, deep breath-out (1, 2, 3, 4, 5, 6).

4. Repeat steps (2) and (3).

Now start your daily affirmation(s) or positive self-talk.

It is also helpful to surround yourself with friends and colleagues who are supportive when you are doing inner work.

MEDITATIVE-RITUALISTIC PRACTICE AND BREATHWORK

There are many different forms of Meditation. Some aim to deepen the mind–body connection, stay present, strengthen feelings of compassion and promote inner peace. Almost all Meditations focus on Breathwork to access our innate healing power. The 'Invitation to Return Home' is a good example of a meditative practice. Yoga, Qi Gong and Tai Chi are examples of movement Meditation where the Breathwork and movements connect the body and mind. These are examples of how we can be in touch with the healing energies of the archaic (Zhi) spirit of the Water element, the magical (Po) spirit of the Metal element and the mythical (Shen) of the Fire element. Participating in a tea ceremony can be said to be a form of spiritual Meditation and ritualistic healing that connects us to the magical (Po Soul) consciousness.

Ritualistic tea ceremony: connecting with the magical (Po Soul) and mythical (Shen)

I knew very little about tea ceremonies until I experienced one with a devoted practitioner of this ancient practice. I am sharing this beautiful experience here because its mindful ritual serves to remind me to slow down, to take in the beauty and connect with our magical (Po Soul) and mythical (Shen) consciousness.

On a lovely Spring afternoon, I had my first experience of a tea ceremony. The Master of the tea ceremony invited me to share a tea ceremony (albeit a modified version) with her under a beautiful old oak tree. I watched as she sat on her heels, paused, breathed, and began the ritual of a tea ceremony. She laid out a runner and gently placed two beautiful small tea bowls on it. I took several slow, deep breaths in and breaths out. I felt myself unwinding; I heard the birds singing, the sun on my back and a gentle breeze stroking my face. I sank into myself and then floated. She ceremoniously rinsed the tea bowls with the hot water with a rotating action. She paused again before bringing a container of tea towards her Heart area, an act of bringing love to the ceremony and its participants. She put a small amount of tea and then the hot water into each bowl. She offered me the tea. I imbibed it slowly, consciously and gratefully and enjoyed every sip. The tea had an agreeable soft taste and a faint flowery fragrance that reminded me of my mother's tea.

As I was witnessing and participating in this tea ceremony, I went into a meditative state and experienced a profound sense of contentment. I was in the flow. I felt a deep sense of connection with myself, the environment and the Master of the tea ceremony. I was grateful to her for making the space and time as well as the warm rays of the sun, gentle breeze and bird song. It was a beautiful embodiment of a spiritual experience that reinforced for me the importance of integrating the meditative, mindful and ritualistic aspects into my daily life.

For centuries, Zen monks, Taoists and Shamans have relied on tea for its medicinal and spiritual power and healing abilities. In the tea ceremony ritual, a sacred space is created in which we sit in silence, turn inward and reconnect to our body, heart and nature, as well as experience the love and gratitude for the simple moments in life. This practice was almost forgotten as tea began to be grown and sold as a commodity. We would be very much impoverished if such rituals were lost. In fact, we can create healing rituals for ourselves in small ways every day – with our daily cup of tea or coffee.

TAI CHI AND QI GONG

The mind–body–spirit practices of Qi Gong and Tai Chi are two of several branches of Chinese medicine. These practices were developed to optimize the Qi (energy) within our body–mind–spirit. They are the foundation of Chinese martial arts that date back thousands of years. Breathwork and mindfulness are essential to these practices that connect to our archaic (Zhi) spirit and magical (Po) soul.

In most forms of Qi Gong, especially active Qi Gong, controlled slow, long, deep abdominal breathing is incorporated into gentle, smooth movements, the aim being to regulate the body–mind–spirit. Additionally, the focus of attention on an intention and visualization is another pillar of Qi Gong. Meditative Qi Gong focuses more on Breathwork and the mind with little body movement.

Tai Chi also involves integrating controlled Breathwork into flowing and focused physical movements. The movements are rather elegant, in my opinion.

The frequent and consistent practice of Qi Gong and Tai Chi has been found to be beneficial in conditions such as sleep disturbance and back pain as well as improving mental function, balance and quality of life in people with chronic illnesses.

New to Qi Gong and Tai Chi? Again, the best way to find an experienced teacher is to ask for recommendations from friends and relatives. Learning Qi Gong or Tai Chi from a video or book does not ensure you are practising the movements and Breathwork correctly.

YOGA AND BREATHWORK
Yoga: connecting with the archaic, magical and mythical consciousness

The practice of Yoga is an excellent way to improve physical and emotional wellbeing as well as providing us with a conduit to connect with the archaic, magical and mythical consciousness. It is useful to know that there are different types of Yoga, including: Power Yoga, Hot Yoga, Flow Yoga, Ashtanga Yoga, Restorative Yoga and Yin Yoga.

All Yoga involves Breathwork. Slow and deep breathing or diaphragmatic breathing can help relax tight muscles and increase flexibility and blood flow. For those in pain, stressed or recuperating from an acute illness, I find the two most suitable are Yin and Restorative Yoga. Before you go to a Yoga class, have an in-depth discussion of what your needs are with the Yoga teacher.

Yin Yoga

Yin Yoga is slow-paced, deceptively difficult and deeply relaxing. This is because you hold certain Yoga poses for longer than that required by other styles of Yoga – anywhere from 3 to 7 minutes. It is always accompanied by Breathwork. For most people the internal chatter ceases while holding a Yin Yoga pose, having arrived at a still and quiet point. You are ready to relax into the pose, and connect with the power and wisdom of the magical structure of consciousness by feeling and listening carefully to your bodily sensations and deep inner knowing. Notice what it feels like to quiet and still, as your body, mind and spirit connect and respond to the Breathwork and the stillness in a pose.

It is believed that regular practice of Yin Yoga helps with joint flexibility, and keeps the fascia, ligaments, tendons and muscles healthy. Equally important, practising Yin Yoga correctly is also an excellent way to prevent and deactivate trigger points.

Restorative Yoga

This is a passive (without active movement or stretch), gentle and meditative Yoga with the emphasis on Breathwork to release deeply held tension. Thus most people find Restorative Yoga relaxing and harmonizing. Restorative Yoga poses are usually 5–10 minutes long, during which time the mind and body are encouraged to relax, and rest deeply and completely. Restorative Yoga is suitable for someone who leads a stressful life, is rehabilitating after a long illness or dealing with a chronic condition. I often recommend Restorative Yoga to my patients, and many of them find this very helpful in dealing with their pain.

Yogic Breathwork

DIAPHRAGMATIC BREATHING

Diaphragmatic breathing, in which the abdomen expands outward during inhalation, can enhance digestion and peristalsis. It triggers the relaxation responses, calming our body and mind, and connecting us to the archaic and magical consciousness. I love this practice. Just like the slow and even Breathwork, it can be practised anywhere, anytime.

1. Begin by getting comfortable.

2. Place one hand over the heart area and the other just below the belly button. (When in a public place, if you do not wish to be too conspicuous, you can cross your arms over the upper abdomen and breathe slowly into the area under the arms and feel your abdomen rise and fall.)

3. Gently lower your eyes.

4. Set an intention to do this breathing.

5. Now focus your attention on your intention to take a breath-in and a breath-out.

6. Take a slow, even and long, deep breath-in to expand the chest and abdomen. Count 1, 2, 3, 4, 5 with each breath-in, feeling the expansion of your diaphragm.

7. Slowly pull your abdominal muscle to the spine, and count 1, 2, 3, 4, 5, 6, as you breathe out. A longer breath helps to empty your lungs and further calms the nervous system, and mind–body.

8. Notice subtle changes in your body and mind. Observe with love, kindness and compassion.

ALTERNATE NOSTRIL BREATHING

I really like the alternate nostril breathing technique too. In my clinic, I often come across patients who are shallow breathers who find it a challenge to do a deep breath-in and breath-out. I observed that they breathe deeper and slower after I've shown them the alternate nostril breathing technique. As the name implies, you alternate each breath-in and breath-out with one nostril and then the other.

Note: The right thumb and right pinky are active (if you prefer to use your left hand, then your left thumb and left pinky are active), the thumb to seal the right nostril and the pinky to seal the left nostril by gently pressing into the nostril.

Here is how to do alternate nostril breathing:

1. This Breathwork is usually done sitting comfortably, cross-leg-ged on the floor. But if this is not your usual practice, find a comfortable, seated position.

2. Take a couple of inhales and exhales before you start.

3. Set your intention to complete this Breathwork.

4. Now focus your attention on your intention.

5. Right thumb to right nostril, inhaling left (for 1, 2, 3, 4, 5), pause.

6. Right pinky to left nostril, exhaling right (for 1, 2, 3, 4, 5, 6), and inhaling right (for 1, 2, 3, 4, 5), pause.

7. Right thumb to right nostril, exhaling left (for 1, 2, 3, 4, 5, 6), pause.

This is one full round. You can stop here, or you can do a few rounds and adjust the number of rounds as desired.

UJJAYI BREATHING

Ujjayi breathing is slow and deep and is believed to be especially effective in activating the parasympathetic nervous system, which is responsible for relaxing the body and helps with the digestive process. When I first started doing Ujjayi breathing, I was very self-conscious and acutely aware of the 'funny' sound coming from my throat. However, soon not only did I overcome my self-consciousness, but when I mastered the technique, I enjoyed the practice and reaped its benefits. Ujjayi breathing is also known as 'ocean breathing' as it sounds like the soft sound of the waves rolling ashore and receding. I like this reframing of a 'funny' sound and it gives me endless joy imagining myself on a beach. In Ujjayi breathing, the lips are gently sealed to direct each breath in and out through the nose and the throat. When this happens, a soft 'haaaahh' is created in the throat. So let's begin:

1. Find a comfortable, seated position.

2. Take a couple of breaths in and out before you start.

3. Set your intention to complete this Breathwork.

4. Now focus your attention on your intention.

5. Imagine that you are blowing out a candle softly, not from your lips, but from your throat.

6. Gently close your lips, breathe in (count 1, 2, 3, 4, 5), through your nose allowing the air to pass through your throat.

7. With lips still gently closed, breathe out (count 1, 2, 3, 4, 5, 6), allowing the air to pass through your throat and out of the nose.

There you are. You have done it. When you get better at Ujjayi breathing, you can also visualize yourself by the beach, relaxing and enjoying the sound of the waves.

YAMUNA BODY ROLLING: CONDITIONING THE WHOLE BODY AND CONNECTING TO THE PO SOUL

Yamuna body rolling (YBR) is an excellent and unique whole-body conditioning programme that was created by Yamuna Zake of New York, USA. Because YBR is a body-based practice and accompanied by Breathwork, it connects us to the magical (Po) soul. YBR involves using your bodyweight on specialized balls of different sizes to stimulate the belly of the muscles, their insertions and attachment points, tendons and ligaments throughout the body. Importantly, this routine is accompanied by a slow, deep breath-in and breath-out. This is an essential and important technique to encourage the body to relax and its weight to gently sink into the ball without force or undue pressure. The YBR technique can be used on the hamstring, inner and outer thighs, abdominal muscles, back, lateral aspects of the body, neck and shoulders. YBR addresses problems related to the fascia, trigger points, muscles, tendons and ligaments. The regular practice of YBR benefits our flexibility, circulation and range of motion, and promotes a calm, relaxed state of mind.

YBR balls come in several sizes and are colour-coded. All except the black calf balls can be deflated, which is a great advantage for travel. The gold ball (previously yellow) is the biggest, and the pressure on the body is lowest. It is recommended for beginners and for sensitive areas such as the rib cage and abdomen. Next comes the silver ball (previously red), which is suitable for the lower extremities, and advanced users. The pearl ball (previously green) is smaller and softer, and is suitable for a smaller physique. The black ball is made for areas of the body such as the calf. Lastly, there is the dark blue ball, the smallest of all, which is as hard as the silver ball. This one is for advanced users.

I recommend enrolling with either Yamuna[17] or other YBR teachers[18] to learn how to effectively use the balls. Once you have mastered the technique, YBR can be done on your own.

CONCLUDING COMMENTS

In this chapter, I have included numerous Yang Sheng practices that help us access the different healing energies of the archaic Zhi spirit, magical Po Soul and mythical Shen. Many of my patients found these self-care practices useful in dealing with their chronic pain and to enhance a sense of wellbeing. However, you can create your personal toolbox. It is important to choose practice(s) that you enjoy, and that suit your healthcare need(s) as well as lifestyle. The next step is to create a daily ritual and to focus your intention to commit to using the tools you have chosen. Keep an open mind and heart when trying new things, and enjoy!

FURTHER READING

Dechar, L.E. (2006) *Five Spirits: Alchemical Acupuncture for Psychological and Spiritual Healing.* New York: Green Press Initiative.

Klein, P.J. and Schneider, R. (2019) 'Qigong and tai chi as therapeutic exercise: Survey of systematic reviews and meta-analyses addressing physical health conditions.' *Alternative Therapies in Health and Medicine 25*(5), 48–53. PMID: 31221939.

NIH (National Center for Complementary and Integrative Health) (no date) 'Yoga: What you need to know.' www.nccih.nih.gov/health/yoga-what-you-need-to-know

Suzuki, S. (2013) 'The theory and technique of Yamuna body rolling.' *Journal of Physical Therapy Science 25*(9), 1197–1200, doi: 10.1589/jpts.25.1197.

References

Andres, M.P., Arcoverde, F.V., Souza, C.C., Fernandes, L.F.C., Abrão, M.S. and Kho, R.M. (2020) 'Extrapelvic endometriosis: A systematic review.' *Journal of Minimally Invasive Gynecology 27*(2), 373–389, doi: 10.1016/j.jmig.2019.10.004.

Ahangari, A. (2014) 'Prevalence of chronic pelvic pain among women: An updated review.' *Pain Physician 17*(2), E141–E147.

As-Sanie, S., Kim, J., Schmidt-Wilcke, T., Sundgren, P.C., Clauw, D.J., Napadow, V. and Harris, R.E. (2016) 'Functional connectivity is associated with altered brain chemistry in women with endometriosis-associated chronic pelvic pain.' *The Journal of Pain 17*(1), 1–13, doi: 10.1016/j.jpain.2015.09.008.

Ballard, K., Lowton, K. and Wright, J. (2006) 'What's the delay? A qualitative study of women's experiences of reaching a diagnosis of endometriosis.' *Fertility and Sterility 86*(5), 1296–1301, doi: 10.1016/j.fertnstert.2006.04.054.

Bata, M.S., Al-Ramahi, M., Salhab, A.A., Gharaibeh, M.N. and Schwartz, J. (2006) 'Delay of ovulation by meloxicam in healthy cycling volunteers: A placebo-controlled, double-blind, crossover study.' *Journal of Clinical Pharmacology 46*(8), 925–932, doi: 10.1177/0091270006289483.

Bazot, M. and Daraï, E. (2017) 'Diagnosis of deep endometriosis: Clinical examination, ultrasonography, magnetic resonance imaging, and other techniques.' *Fertility and Sterility 108*(6), 886–894, doi: 10.1016/j.fertnstert.2017.10.026.

Bond, M.R. and Pilowsky, I. (1966) 'Subjective assessment of pain and its relationship to the administration of analgesics in patients with advanced cancer.' *Journal of Psychosomatic Research 10*(2), 203–208, doi: 10.1016/0022-3999(66)90064-x.

Brawn, J., Morotti, M., Zondervan, K.T., Becker, C.M. and Vincent, K. (2014) 'Central changes associated with chronic pelvic pain and endometriosis.'

Human Reproduction Update 20(5), 737–747. https://doi.org/10.1093/humupd/dmu025

Brill, A.I., Nezhat, F., Nezhat, C.H. and Nezhat, C. (1995) 'The incidence of adhesions after prior laparotomy: A laparoscopic appraisal.' *Obstetrics and Gynecology 85*(2), 269–272, doi: 10.1016/0029-7844(94)00352-E.

Bryant, C., Cockburn, R., Plante, A.-F. and Chia, A. (2016) 'The psychological profile of women presenting to a multidisciplinary clinic for chronic pelvic pain: High levels of psychological dysfunction and implications for practice.' *Journal of Pain Research 9*, 1049–1056, doi: 10.2147/JPR.S115065.

Carey, E.T., Till, S.R. and As-Sanie, S. (2017) 'Pharmacological management of chronic pelvic pain in women.' *Drugs 77*(3), 285–301, doi: 10.1007/s40265-016-0687-8.

Chan, S. (2019) 'Sometimes physical pain isn't the worst part about chronic illness.' *A Chronic Voice*, Blog, 7 September. www.achronicvoice.com/2019/09/07/pain-chronic-illness

Chong, O.-T., Critchley, H.O., Horne, A.W., Fallon, M. and Haraldsdottir, E. (2018a) 'Chronic pelvic pain in women: An embedded qualitative study to evaluate the perceived benefits of the meridian balance method electro-acupuncture treatment, health consultation and National Health Service standard care.' *British Journal of Pain 13*(4). https://doi.org/10.1177/2049463718814870

Chong, O.-T., Critchley, H.O., Williams, L.J., Haraldsdottir, E., Horne, A.W. and Fallon, M. (2018b) 'The impact of meridian balance method electro-acupuncture treatment on chronic pelvic pain in women: A three-armed randomised controlled feasibility study using a mixed-methods approach.' *British Journal of Pain 12*(4), 238–249, doi: 10.1177/2049463718776044.

Cornell, A.W. (1996) *The Power of Focusing.* Oakland, CA: New Harbinger Publications, Inc.

Davies, C. and Davies, A. (2013) *The Trigger Point Therapy Workbook: Your Self-Treatment Guide for Pain Relief* (3rd edn). Oakland, CA: New Harbinger Publications, Inc.

Davies, L., Gangar, K.F., Drummond, M., Saunders, D. and Beard, R.W. (1992) 'The economic burden of intractable gynaecological pain.' *Journal of Obstetrics and Gynaecology 12*, S54–S56, doi: 10.3109/01443619209045615.

Deadman, P., Al-Khafaji, M. and Baker, K. (2001) *A Manual of Acupuncture.* Hove: Journal of Chinese Medicine Publications.

Dechar, L.E. (2006) *Five Spirits: Alchemical Acupuncture for Psychological and Spiritual Healing.* New York: Lantern Books.

REFERENCES

Dechar, L.E. (2021) *Kigo: Exploring the Spiritual Essence of Acupuncture Points Through the Changing Seasons.* London: Singing Dragon.

Dechar, L.E. and Fox, B. (2021) *The Alchemy of Inner Work.* Newburyport, MA: Weiser Books.

Dechar, L.E., Fox, B. and Shaw, J. (2020) 'Awakening Consciousness for Healing.' [Online course.] https://community.anewpossibility.com

de Graaff, A.A., D'Hooghe, T.M., Dunselman, G.A.J., Dirksen, C.D., Hummelshoj, L., Werf EndoCost Consortium, Simoens, S., Bokor, A., Brandes, I. and Brodszky, V. (2013) 'The significant effect of endometriosis on physical, mental and social wellbeing: Results from an international cross-sectional survey.' *Human Reproduction 28*(10), 2677–2685, doi: 10.1093/humrep/det284.

Dekker, J., Hooijer, I., Ket, J.C.F., Vejnović, A., Benagiano, G., Brosens, I. and Mijatovic, V. (2021) 'Neonatal uterine bleedings: An ignored sign but a possible cause of early-onset endometriosis – A systematic review.' *Biomedicine Hub 6*(1), 6–16, doi: 10.1159/000512663.

Engeler, D.B., Baranowski, A.P., Berghmans, B., Birch, J., Borovicka, J., Cottrell, A.M., Dinis-Oliveira, P., Elneil, S., Hughes, J., Messelink, E.J., Pinto, R.A., van Poelgeest, M.L., Tidman, V. and de C Williams, A.C. (2022) *EAU Guidelines on Chronic Pelvic Pain.* Arnhem: European Association of Urology Guidelines Office. https://d56bochluxqnz.cloudfront.net/documents/full-guideline/EAU-Guidelines-on-Chronic-Pelvic-Pain-2022_2022-03-29-084111_kpbq.pdf

ESHRE (European Society of Human Reproduction and Embryology) (2022) 'ESHRE Guideline Endometriosis'. 2 February. www.eshre.eu/Guidelines-and-Legal/Guidelines/Endometriosis-guideline

Fall, M., Baranowski, A.P., Elneil, S., Engeler, D., Hughes, J., Messelink, E.J., Oberpenning, F. and de C Williams, A.C. (2010) 'EAU Guidelines on Chronic Pelvic Pain.' *European Urology 57*(1), 35–48, doi: 10.1016/j.eururo.2009.08.020.

Ford, A.C., Lacy, B.E., Harris, L.A., Quigley, E.M.M. and Moayyedi, P. (2019) 'Effect of antidepressants and psychological therapies in irritable bowel syndrome: An updated systematic review and meta-analysis.' *The American Journal of Gastroenterology 114*(1), 21–39, doi: 10.1038/s41395-018-0222-5.

Foster, H.E., Jr, Hanno, P.M., Nickel, J.C., Payne, C.K., Mayer, R.D., Burks, D.A., Yang, C.C., Chai, T.C., Kreder, K.J., Peters, K.M., Lukacz, E.S., Fitzgerald, M.P., Cen, L., Landis, J.R., Propert, K.J., Yang, W., Kusek, J.W. and Nyberg, L.M. (2010) 'Effect of amitriptyline on symptoms in treatment naïve patients with interstitial cystitis/painful bladder syndrome.' *The Journal of Urology 183*(5), 1853–1858, doi: 10.1016/j.juro.2009.12.106.

Francis, C.Y. and Whorwell, P.J. (1994) 'Bran and irritable bowel syndrome: Time for reappraisal.' *The Lancet 344*(8914), 39–40, doi: 10.1016/s0140-6736(94)91055-3.

Grosman-Rimon, L., Parkinson, W., Upadhye, S., Clarke, H., Katz, J., Flannery, J., Peng, P. and Kumbhare, D. (2016) 'Circulating biomarkers in acute myofascial pain: A case-control study.' *Medicine 95*(37), e4650, doi: 10.1097/MD.0000000000004650.

Guo, S.-W. (2009) 'Recurrence of endometriosis and its control.' *Human Reproduction Update 15*(4), 441–461, doi: 10.1093/humupd/dmp007.

Hanno, P.M., Erickson, D., Moldwin, R. and Faraday, M.M. (2015) 'Diagnosis and treatment of interstitial cystitis/bladder pain syndrome: AUA guideline amendment.' *The Journal of Urology 193*, 1545–1553. http://dx.doi.org/10.1016/j.juro.2015.01.086

Horne, A.W. and Saunders, P.T.K. (2019) 'SnapShot: Endometriosis.' *Cell 179*(7), 1677–1677, doi: 10.1016/j.cell.2019.11.033.

Howard, F.M. (2000) 'The role of laparoscopy as a diagnostic tool in chronic pelvic pain.' *Best Practice & Research Clinical Obstetrics & Gynaecology 14*(3), 467–494, doi: 10.1053/beog.1999.0086.

Huang, G., Le, A.-L., Goddard, Y., James, D., Thavorn, K., Payne, M. and Chen, I. (2021) 'A systematic review of the cost of chronic pelvic pain in women.' *Journal of Obstetrics and Gynaecology Canada 44*(3), 286–293, doi: 10.1016/j.jogc.2021.08.011.

Jiang, S. and Zhao, J.-S. (2016) 'The historical source of "Trigger Points": Classical ashi points.' *World Journal of Acupuncture-Moxibustion 26*, 11–14, doi: 10.1016/S1003-5257(17)30003-X.

Johnson, J. (2019) *Seeing Through the World: Jean Gebser and Integral Consiousness*, Seattle, WA: Revelore Press.

Kavuri, V., Selvan, P., Malamud, A., Raghuram, N. and Selvan, S.R. (2015) 'Remedial yoga module remarkably improves symptoms in irritable bowel syndrome patients: A 12-week randomized controlled trial.' *European Journal of Integrative Medicine 7*(6), 595–608. https://doi.org/10.1016/j.eujim.2015.11.001

Khanna, R., MacDonald, J.K. and Levesque, B.G. (2014) 'Peppermint oil for the treatment of irritable bowel syndrome: A systematic review and meta-analysis.' *Journal of Clinical Gastroenterology 48*(6), 505–512, doi: 10.1097/MCG.0b013e3182a88357.

REFERENCES

Laganà, A.S., La Rosa, V.L., Rapisarda, A.M.C., Valenti, G., Sapia, F., Chiofalo, B., Rossetti, D., Ban Frangež, H., Vrtačnik Bokal, E. and Vitale, S.G. (2017) 'Anxiety and depression in patients with endometriosis: Impact and management challenges.' *International Journal of Women's Health 9*, 323–330, doi: 10.2147/IJWH.S119729.

Laux-Biehlmann, A., D'Hooghe, T. and Zollner, T.M. (2015) 'Menstruation pulls the trigger for inflammation and pain in endometriosis.' *Trends in Pharmacological Sciences 36*(5), 270–276, doi: 10.1016/j.tips.2015.03.004.

Mu, F., Harris, H.R., Rich-Edwards, J.W., Hankinson, S.E., Rimm, E.B., Spiegelman, D. and Missmer, S.A. (2018) 'A prospective study of inflammatory markers and risk of endometriosis.' *American Journal of Epidemiology 187*(3), 515–522, doi: 10.1093/aje/kwx272.

NICE (National Institute for Health and Care Excellence) (2008) Irritable Bowel Syndrome in Adults: Diagnosis and Management. Clinical Guideline 61. [Updated 4 April 2017.] www.nice.org.uk/Guidance/CG61

NICE (National Institute for Health and Care Excellence) (2021) Chronic Pain (Primary and Secondary) in Over 16s: Assessment of All Chronic Pain and Management of Chronic Primary Pain. NICE Guideline 193. www.nice. org.uk/ng193

Nnoaham, K.E., Hummelshoj, L., Webster, P., D'Hooghe, T., de Cicco Nardone, F., de Cicco Nardone, C., Jenkinson, C., Kennedy, S.H. and Zondervan, K.T. (2011) 'Impact of endometriosis on quality of life and work productivity: A multicenter study across ten countries.' *Fertility and Sterility 96*(2), 366–373, doi: 10.1016/j.fertnstert.2011.05.090.

O'Hare, P.G., 3rd, Hoffmann, A.R., Allen, P., Gordon, B., Salin, L. and Whitmore, K. (2013) 'Interstitial cystitis patients' use and rating of complementary and alternative medicine therapies.' *International Urogynecology Journal 24*(6), 977–982, doi: 10.1007/s00192-012-1966-x.

Prescott, J., Farland, L.V., Tobias, D.K., Gaskins, A.J., Spiegelman, D., Chavarro, J.E., Rich-Edwards, J.W., Barbieri, R.L. and Missmer, S.A. (2016) 'A prospective cohort study of endometriosis and subsequent risk of infertility.' *Human Reproduction 31*(7), 1475–1482. https://doi.org/10.1093/humrep/dew085

RCOG (Royal College of Obstetricians and Gynaecologists) (2016) Management of Bladder Pain Syndrome. Green-top Guideline No. 70. www. rcog.org.uk/guidance/browse-all-guidance/green-top-guidelines/ management-of-bladder-pain-syndrome-green-top-guideline-no-70

Saunders, P.T.K. and Horne, A.W. (2021) 'Endometriosis: Etiology, pathobiology, and therapeutic prospects.' *Cell 184*(11), 2807–2824, doi: 10.1016/j.cell.2021.04.041.

Schwartz, E.S. and Gebhart, G.F. (2014) 'Visceral pain.' In B. Taylor and D. Finn (eds) *Behavioral Neurobiology of Chronic Pain: Current Topics in Behavioral Neurosciences*, vol. 20 (pp.171–197). Berlin, Heidelberg: Springer. https://doi.org/10.1007/7854_2014_315

Seem, M. (1993) *A New American Acupuncture-Myofasical Release of the Bodymind's Holding Patterns.* Boulder, CO: Blue Poppy Press.

Shafrir, A.L., Farland, L.V., Shah, D.K., Harris, H.R., Kvaskoff, M., Zondervan, K. and Missmer, S.A. (2018) 'Risk for and consequences of endometriosis: A critical epidemiologic review.' *Best Practice & Research Clinical Obstetrics & Gynaecology 51*, 1–15, doi: 10.1016/j.bpobgyn.2018.06.001.

Simoens, S., Hummelshoj, L., Dunselman, G., Brandes, I., Dirksen, C., D'Hooghe, T. and EndoCost Consortium (2011) 'Endometriosis cost assessment (the EndoCost study): A cost-of-illness study protocol.' *Gynecologic and Obstetric Investigation 71*(3), 170–176, doi: 10.1159/000316055.

Simons, D.G., Travell, J.G. and Simons, L.S. (1999) *Myofascial Pain and Dysfunction: The Trigger Point Manual. Vol. 1: Upper Half of the Body* (2nd edn). Baltimore, MD: Lippincott, Williams & Wilkins.

Tan, R.T.-F. (2003) *Dr Tan's Strategy of Twelve Magical Points.* San Diego, CA: Richard Tan.

Thilagarajah, R., Witherow, R.O. and Walker, M.M. (2001) 'Oral cimetidine gives effective symptom relief in painful bladder disease: A prospective, randomized, double-blind placebo-controlled trial.' *BJU International 87*(3), 207–212, doi: 10.1046/j.1464-410x.2001.02031.x.

Thornton, M., Campeau, J. and Dizerega, G. (1997) 'Use of Adhesion Prevention Barriers in Gynecological Surgery.' In K.-H. Treutner and V. Schumpelick (eds) *Peritoneal Adhesions* (pp.370–385). Cham: Springer.

Tirlapur, S.A., Kuhrt, K., Chaliha, C., Ball, E., Meads, C. and Khan, K.S. (2013) 'The "evil twin syndrome" in chronic pelvic pain: A systematic review of prevalence studies of bladder pain syndrome and endometriosis.' *International Journal of Surgery 11*(3), 233–237, doi: 10.1016/j.ijsu.2013.02.003.

Tracey, I. (2016) 'Finding the hurt in pain.' *Cerebrum.* www.ncbi.nlm.nih.gov/pmc/articles/PMC5501013

Travell, J.G. and Simons, D.G. (1993) *Myofascial Pain and Dysfunction: The Trigger Point Manual. Vol. 2: The Lower Extremities* (2nd edn). Philadephia, PA: Lippincott Williams & Wilkins.

REFERENCES

Tripoli, T.M., Sato, H., Sartori, M.G., de Araujo, F.F., Girão, M.J.B.C. and Schor, E. (2011) 'Evaluation of quality of life and sexual satisfaction in women suffering from chronic pelvic pain with or without endometriosis.' *The Journal of Sexual Medicine 8*(2), 497–503, doi: 10.1111/j.1743-6109.2010.01976.x.

Tu, F.F., As-Sanie, S. and Steege, J.F. (2006) 'Prevalence of pelvic musculoskeletal disorders in a female chronic pelvic pain clinic.' *The Journal of Reproductive Medicine 51*(3), 185–189.

Vercellini, P., Trespidi, L., Colombo, A., Vendola, N., Marchini, M. and Crosignani, P.G. (1993) 'A gonadotropin-releasing hormone agonist versus a low-dose oral contraceptive for pelvic pain associated with endometriosis.' *Fertility and Sterility 60*(1), 75–79. https://doi.org/10.1016/S0015-0282(16)56039-7

Warren, J.W., Brown, J., Tracy, J.K., Langenberg, P., Wesselmann, U. and Greenberg, P. (2008) 'Evidence-based criteria for pain of interstitial cystitis/painful bladder syndrome in women.' *The Journal of Urology 71*(3), 444–448, doi: 10.1016/j.urology.2007.10.062.

Weiss, J.M. (2019) *Breaking Through Chronic Pelvic Pain: A Holistic Approach for Relief.* Jerome M. Weiss.

Woolf, C.J. (2011) 'Central sensitization: Implications for the diagnosis and treatment of pain.' *Pain 152*(3 Suppl.), S2–S15, doi: 10.1016/j.pain.2010.09.030.

Zondervan, K.T. and Barlow, D.H. (2000) 'Epidemiology of chronic pelvic pain.' *Best Practice & Research Clinical Obstetrics & Gynaecology 14*(3), 403–414, doi: 10.1053/beog.1999.0083.

Zondervan, K.T., Yudkin, P.L., Vessey, M.P., Dawes, M.G., Barlow, D.H. and Kennedy, S.H. (1999) 'Prevalence and incidence of chronic pelvic pain in primary care: Evidence from a national general practice database.' *BJOG: An International Journal of Obstetrics & Gynaecology 106*(11), 1149–1155, doi: 10.1111/j.1471-0528.1999.tb08140.x.

Zondervan, K.T., Yudkin, P.L., Vessey, M.P., Jenkinson, C.P., Dawes, M.G., Barlow, D.H. and Kennedy, S.H. (2001) 'Chronic pelvic pain in the community – Symptoms, investigations, and diagnoses.' *American Journal of Obstetrics and Gynecology 184*(6), 1149–1155, doi: 10.1067/mob.2001.112904.

Endnotes

1   I needled the Ashi points around the Hand Yang Ming/LI 4 and Hand Yang Ming/LI 10–11 on the left side (the opposite side to her pain). She identified the area of most pain in the right lower abdomen, around the Stomach/Foot Yang Ming meridian.

2   Reiki is a healing technique that is based on the notion that the therapist can channel energy into the patient by vibrational touch to activate the healing process and restore physical and emotional wellbeing.

3   I based this practice on my clinical experience. I noticed that when I held a patient's heels with my hands and breathed with them, they quickly fell into a deep relaxation state. Patients often commented that they felt very safe and grounded with this hands-on treatment. Later I realized that what I was doing was accessing the archaic energy, our powerful healing source that is related to the Water element. The Kidney and Bladder meridians travel along the inner and outer malleolus, down to the heels and outer aspects of the feet.

4   NICE is a public body that provides national guidance and advice that is evidenced based. It is funded by the Department of Health and Social Care, UK.

5   Dr Eileen Han, Balance Method acupuncture: https://eileenhan.com and Dr Delphine Armand, Si Yuan Balance Method: www.siyuanbalance.com (both Dr Han and Dr Armand studied closely (as disciples) with Dr Tan).

6   Dr Richard Tan's lecture series 'The Balance Method', New York, September 2008 and October 2009.

7   Dr Richard Tan's lecture series 'The Balance Method', London, July 2015.

8   Sometimes called the *I Ching*. It is one of the oldest Chinese classical texts, which was created in the Western Zhou period (1000–750 BC). It is believed to be the work of Fu Shi (2852 BC) who proposed how the universe was

formed and its relationship to human beings through his observation of the seasons, day and night, and the movements of the sun, moon and stars. The Taiji (Yin–Yang theory) and the Five Elements cycle originated in the *Yi Ching* and importantly form the basis for the entire theory of Chinese medicine, including BM acupuncture taught by Dr Tan. The Five Elements cycle is associated with the eight trigrams that feature prominently in BM acupuncture.

9   The Chinese energy clock is another important tool in Chinese medicine. It is based on the notion that it is most advantageous to treat the organ when its energy is at its peak. For example, the lungs' energy is at its peak between 3 am and 5 am, and so this is the time to treat them. The Chinese energy clock can be likened to the circadian rhythm.

10 See, for example, www.triggerpoints.nets, https://twitter.com/i/events/1440588296048889859,www.pinterest.com/pin/476044623092447209

11 See https://classicalchinesemedicine.org/healing-through-the-emotions-the-confucian-therapy-system-of-wang-fengyi

12 Lorie and her husband, Benjamin Fox, created A New Possibility, a learning and healing community for both professionals and laypeople. For in-depth learning in these techniques, please enrol in the courses offered on their website at https://anewpossibility.com

13 See https://mentorship.healthyseminars.com/members/lorie-eve-dechar

14 I learned these through my participation in Lorie Eve Dechar and Benjamin Fox's 'Alchemical Healing Mentorship' in 2009.

15 'Chinese Dietary Therapy', August 2007, New York, USA. Dr Jeffrey Yuen is a highly respected teacher and practitioner of classical Chinese medicine. He is 88th Generation Daoist Master of the Jade Purity School.

16 My opinion is that the 'Spleen' has been mistranslated. I believe that the 'Spleen' really refers to the 'Pancreas'. However, we are stuck with the term 'Spleen'.

17 www.yamunausa.com

18 https://yamunabodyrolling.co.uk

Index

abandonment fear 22
abdominal muscles trigger points 107–11
abuse (history of) 26, 147
acrid flavour 169
acupuncture (overview) 38–9
adductor magnus muscles
    trigger points 112–3
adhesions (pain from) 30–1
affirmations 123, 129, 191–3
Aggressive Energy treatment 134–7
Ahangari, A. 15
Al-Khafaji, M. 84, 107, 145
Alchemical Healing
  benevolent dragon 150–1
  breathwork/visualization in 146
  case study 19, 21–2
  fear/anger to wisdom/
    compassion 149–52
  golden key 146–7
  healing power of point names 147–8
  initial acupuncture treatment 145–6
  overview 143–4
  patient examples 144–52
  point selection 151–2
  psychic and emotional pain 144–9
  ritual creation 148, 160
alternate nostril breathing 197–8
amitriptyline 34, 37
amplification 30–1
anatomical similarity 66
Andres, M.P. 28
anger (Wood personality) 124–5
animal symbols (Five Elements) 119
anticoagulants 102

antidepressants 32–3
anxiety 20, 21–2, 144–5
archaic structure 152, 154
archetypes 120, 191–2
arrogance (Water personality) 121–2
As-Sanie, S. 29, 30, 95
Ashi points 46–7, 95
Autumn 169

Ba Gua (hexagram) 75, 76–81
Baker, K. 84, 107, 145
Balance Method see Global Balance
    Method; Local Balance Method
Ballard, K. 27
Barlow, D.H. 40
Bata, M.S. 36
Bazot, M. 28
beans 167, 171
benevolent dragon 137–9, 150–1
Biao-Li/interior–exterior pairs
    49–50, 55–6, 63, 64
Bie-Jing/branching meridians
    48–9, 54–5, 63, 64
Biel, Andrew 96
bitter flavour 165, 167
black sesame seeds 170
blame (Earth personality) 130
BM acupuncture case studies 17–8
Bond, M.R. 97
branching meridians 48–9, 54–5, 63, 64
Brawn, J. 30
Breathwork
  alternate nostril breathing 197–8
  diaphragmatic breathing 197

213

Breathwork *cont.*
  slow 187–8
  Ujjayi breathing 198–9
  and visualization 146, 188–9
Brill, A.I. 30
Bryant, C. 41

Campeau, J. 31
Carey, E.T. 29
case studies
  Biao-Li/interior–exterior
    pairs 55–6, 63, 64
  Bie-Jing/branching meridians
    54–5, 63, 64
  Chinese meridian name sharing 53–4
  complex pain 62–5
  Five Elements 139–40
  image method 54, 56, 58, 60–1, 63, 65
  image method (in-depth study) 60–1
  impact of living with chronic
    pelvic pain 40
  mirror method 53–4, 56, 58, 59
central sensitization 30–1
Chan, S. 15
childhood abuse 147
Chinese clock neighbours
  51, 58–60, 63, 64
Chinese clock opposites 50–1, 56–8, 63,
  64
Chinese meridian name sharing
  48, 53–4, 63, 64
Chong, O.-T. 41, 42, 45, 135
chronic pelvic pain
  causes 25–6
  definition 25
  prevalence 15
  see also endometriosis; impact of
    living with chronic pelvic pain
cimetidine 34
citrus fruits 166
coccygeus muscle 103
coffee 167
cognitive behavioural therapy 33
colours of Five Elements 118, 121–2,
  124, 130, 139, 166–71
complex pain 62–5
connection 126
consciousness see Gebser's theory
  of consciousness

cooked vs. raw food 172–3
Cornell, A.W. 157
cross-organ sensitization pain 30

dandelion greens 171
Daraï, E. 28
dark chocolate 167
Davies, A. 93, 94, 96, 103
Davies, C. 93, 94, 96, 103
Davies, L. 42
de Graaff, A.A. 41
Deadman, P. 84, 107, 145
Dechar, L.E. 18, 22, 118, 143,
  146, 152, 156, 175
deep endometriosis (DE) 28
Dekker, J. 27
depression 20, 144–5
D'Hooghe, T. 29
digestive system
  overview 164–5
  Spleen functions 177–8
  Stomach functions 177–8
Dizerega, G. 31
doing by not doing (Wu Wei) 158–9
dry needling 96–7
dualism 153
Dynamic Balance 73–4, 86–91

Earth archetype 192
Earth personality 129–31
Eight Magical Points treatment 82
emotions of Five Elements 118,
  121–2, 124–5, 127, 130
endometrioma 28
endometriosis
  causes 27
  diagnosis 27
  and fertility 27
  lesions 28
  overview 26–7
  symptoms 26–7
  treatment 36–8
  types of 28
  types of pain associated with 29–31
'energetics of food' 171–2
Engeler, D.B. 26
ESHRE (European Society of
  Human Reproduction and
  Embryology) 36, 38

— 214 —

INDEX

evil Qi 134–7
EXPPECT Centre for Pelvic Pain and Endometriosis 38–9
External Dragons treatment 137–9

Fall, M. 33
fascia 94
fatigue 42
fear 21–2, 121–2, 149–52
feedback from patients 66
'felt sense' 157
fertility 27
financial burden 42
Fire archetype 191–2
Fire personality 126–9
Five Elements
　acupuncture treatment 133–40
　associations 118–9
　case study 139–40
　Earth element 118–9, 165
　Fire element 118–9, 165, 167
　flavours 165–71
　Metal element 118–9, 165, 169
　overview 117–8
　treatment protocols 134–9
　Water element 118–9, 165, 170–1
　Wood element 118–9, 165, 166
five flavours 119, 165–6
Five Shu points 83–5
Five Systems
　System 1 Chinese meridian name sharing 48, 53–4, 63, 64
　System 2 Bie-Jing/branching meridians 48–9, 54–5, 63, 64
　System 3 Biao-Li/interior–exterior pairs 49–50, 55–6, 63, 64
　System 4 Chinese clock opposites 50–1, 56–8, 63, 64
　System 5 Chinese clock neighbours 51, 58–60, 63, 64
flavour of Five Elements 119, 165–71
Flaws, B. 180
food
　cooking vs. raw 172–3
　enjoyment of 175
　Yin–Yang spectrum 171–2
food elimination method 34
Ford, A.C. 33
Foster, H.E. 34

Fox, B. 143, 152
Francis, C.Y. 32
frequency of treatment 67

gabapentin 37
Gebhart, G.F. 30
Gebser's theory of consciousness
　archaic structure 152, 154
　magical structure 152, 154–5, 157–8
　mythical structure 153, 155–6
Gendlin, Eugene 157
Global Balance Method
　Dynamic Balance 73–4, 86–91
　Eight Magical Points treatment 82
　meridian conversion 75–81
　Static Balance 70–3, 78–82
　three-step algorithm 74–5
　Twelve Magical Points treatment 82–5, 88–91
gonadotropin-releasing hormone agonists (GnRHa) 36–7
grains 168
grief (Metal personality) 132
Grosman-Rimon, L. 95
Guo, S.-W. 37
gut feeling 132, 154–5, 157

Han, Eileen Yue-Ling 46
Hanno, P.M. 33
harmonious personality 121
hate (Fire personality) 127
He Sea points 76, 83–5, 86
Heart space 128, 144, 155, 159
hexagram (Ba Gua) 75, 76–81
hormonal suppression therapies 36–7
Horne, A.W. 26, 27, 28
Howard, F.M. 26
Huang, G. 42
Hun spirit 125
hypnotherapy 33

iliopsoas muscle trigger points 113–5
image method
　case studies 54, 55, 56, 58, 60–1, 63
　overview 52–3
　point selection 85–6
impact of living with chronic pelvic pain
　case report 40
　overview 40–1

impact of living with chronic
pelvic pain *cont.*
  personal/societal cost 42
  sexual wellbeing/intimacy 41
inflammatory pain 29
Inner Sensing 157–8
insoluble fibre 32
integral structure 156
intention 159, 186
interior–exterior pairs 49–50, 55–6, 63, 64
Internal Dragons treatment 137–8, 150–1
intimacy/sexual wellbeing 41
intuition 132, 154–5, 157
'Invitation to Return Home'
  exercise 20–1, 146
irritable bowel syndrome (IBS) 31–3

Jiang, S. 95
Jing River points 76, 83–5, 86, 88
Jing Well points 76, 83–5, 86, 87
Johnson, J. 119, 144
joy (Fire personality) 127
judgement (Metal personality) 132
Jung, Carl 120, 155

Kavuri, V. 32
Khanna, R. 32

Lagana, A.S. 39
laparoscopy 27
Laux-Biehlmann, A. 29
levator ani 103
Levesque, B.G. 32
lidocaine 34
listening to the patient 66–7
Local Balance Method
  evidence for 45
  image method 52–3, 54, 56,
    58, 60–1, 63, 65
  mirror method 52, 53–4, 56, 58, 59
  overview 45–7
  reverse image method 53
  three-step algorithm 47, 61, 62–4
  using the Five Systems 47–51
logic 131–2
love 126
lower rectus abdominis trigger
  points 108–10

Lowton, K. 27
Lu, H.C. 163

MacDonald, J.K. 32
magical structure 152, 154–5, 157–8
marital problems 41
matrix analysis 62–5
mealtimes (optimal) 176
medications
  amitriptyline 34, 37
  antidepressants 32–3
  cimetidine 34
  endometriosis 36
  hormonal suppression therapies 36–7
  irritable bowel syndrome (IBS) 32–3
  lidocaine 34
  neuromodulators 37
  non-steroidal anti-inflammatory
    drugs (NSAIDs) 36
meditative-ritualistic practice 193–4
mental structure 153
meridian conversion
  overview 75–7
  Shao Yang–Tai Yin pattern 80–1
  Tai Yin–Yang Ming pattern 78–80
meridian name sharing 48, 63, 64
meridians
  in Dynamic Balance 73–4, 86–91
  in Static Balance 70–3
Metal archetype 192
Metal personality 131–3
mirror method 52, 53–4, 56, 58, 59
Mu, F. 29
myofascial pain syndrome 35
mythical structure 153, 155–6

narrative (changing) 190
needling technique 100–1, 135, 139
negative self-talk 189–90, 193
neuromodulators 37
neuropathic pain 29
NICE (National Institute for Health
  and Care Excellence) 31
Nnoaham, K.E. 27
nociceptive pain 29
non-steroidal anti-inflammatory
  drugs (NSAIDs) 36
nourishing/nurturing personality 129
nuts 169

INDEX

oblique muscles 110–1
obturator internus 104–5
oestrogen therapy 36–7
O'Hare, P.G. 34
'one bowl eating meditation' 175–6
onion family 169
organs of Five Elements 118
ovarian endometriosis (endometrioma) 28

pain
  complex 62–5
  cross-organ sensitization 30
  from adhesions 30–1
  inflammatory 29
  menstrual 36
  neuropathic 29
  nociceptive 29
  in painful bladder syndrome (PBS) 33
  visual analogue scale (VAS) 97–8
painful bladder syndrome (PBS) 33–5
panic attacks 20
pelvic diaphragm 103
pelvic floor muscles trigger points 102–7
peppermint oil 32
personal/societal cost 42
personality/temperament
  Earth personality 129–31
  Fire personality 126–9
  Metal personality 131–3
  overview 120
  Water personality 121–3
  Wood personality 123–6
physiotherapy 39
Pilowsky, I. 97
piriformis muscle 105–7
Pitchford, P. 163
Po Soul 132–3
point names (healing power
  of) 147–8, 159–60
point selection
  Aggressive Energy treatment 136
  in Alchemical Healing 145–6,
    147–8, 151–2, 159–60
  External Dragons treatment 138
  image method 52–3, 54, 56, 58,
    60–1, 63, 65, 85–6
  Internal Dragons treatment 138
  mirror method 52, 53–4, 56, 58, 59
  Shao Yang–Tai Yin pattern 81

Tai Yin–Yang Ming pattern 78–80
power of Five Elements 119
precision 131–2
pregabalin 37
pregnant patients 102
Prescott, J. 27
primary chronic pain 26
progestogen therapy 36–7
psycho-emotional pain see
  Alchemical Healing
psychological approaches 39
pulses 166
pungent flavour 169

Qi Gong 195
qualities of Five Elements 119

raw vs. cooked food 172–3
RCOG (Royal College of Obstetricians
  and Gynaecologists) 33
relationship problems 41, 42
restorative Yoga 196
retrograde menstruation theory 27
reverse image method 53, 85, 86
rice 168
ritual creation 148, 160
ritualistic tea ceremony 193–4
roots 169

salty flavour 166, 170–1
Saunders, P.T.K. 26, 27, 28
Schwartz, E.S. 30
seasons of Five Elements 118,
  126, 166, 167, 169, 170
seaweed 170
seeds 167, 169, 170
Seem, M. 96, 97
self-talk 189–90, 193
Seven Dragons treatment 137–9
sexual dysfunction 41
Shao Yang–Tai Yin pattern 80–1
Shaw, J. 152
Shen spirit 20, 128, 144, 159
shopping mindfully 173–4
Shu Stream points 76, 83–5, 86, 87, 88
Simoens, S. 42
Simons, D.G. 15, 96, 113
Simons, L.S. 15, 96
sleep disturbances 42

social isolation 42
societal cost 42
soluble fibre 32
sounds of Five Elements 118
sour flavour 165, 166
sphincter ani 103
spicy flavour 166, 169
spirits of Five Elements 118, 119–20
Spleen digestive functions 177–8
Spleen Qi deficiency 179
Spleen Yang deficiency 180
Spring 166
Static Balance 70–3, 78–82
Steege, J.F. 95
Stomach Cold 179–80
Stomach digestive functions 177–8
Stomach Heat/Fire 181
Stomach Qi deficiency 178
Stomach Yin deficiency 181–2
stress management (PBS) 34
structural imbalance 46
Summer 126, 167
sunflower seeds 170
superficial peritoneal
        endometriosis (SPE) 28
surgery (for endometriosis) 37–8
sweet/bland flavour 165, 167–9
sympathy (Earth personality) 130

Tai Chi 195
Tai Yin–Yang Ming pattern 78–80
Tan, R.T.-F. 46, 69
tea 167
tea ceremony 193–4
temperament see personality/temperament
Thilagarajah, R. 34
Thornton, M. 31
three-step algorithm 47, 61, 62–4
Till, S.R. 29
Tirlapur, S.A. 33
Tracey, I. 30
Travell, J.G. 15, 96, 113
trigger point deactivation
    abdominal muscles trigger
        points 107–11
    adductor magnus muscles
        trigger points 112–3
    classical approach to 96–7
    contraindications/precautions 101–2

iliopsoas muscle trigger points 113–5
needling instructions 100–1
pelvic floor muscles trigger points 102–7
preparation of healthcare
        professional 99–100
preparation of patient 97–9
trigger points (overview) 93–6
Tripoli, T.M. 41
Tu, F.F. 95
Twelve Magical Points treatment
        82–5, 88–91
twitch response 93, 97, 98–9

Ujjayi breathing 198–9
undereating 176
upper rectus abdominis trigger
        points 108–10
urogenital diaphragm 103

vegetables 166, 167, 169
Vercellini, P. 37
virtues of Five Elements 118
visual analogue scale (VAS) 97–8
visualization 146, 186–7, 188–9

Walker, M.M. 34
Wang Fengyi 117
Warren, J.W. 34
Water archetype 192
Water personality 121–3
Weiss, J.M. 107
Western medical model 153
Whorwell, P.J. 32
Winter 170
Witherow, R.O. 34
Wood archetype 191
Wood personality 123–6
Woolf, C.J. 30
work lives 42
Worsley, J.R. 133
Wright, J. 27
Wu Wei 158–9

Xie Qi 134–5

Yamuna body rolling (YBR) 199–200
Yang meridians 76
Yang Sheng 185

INDEX

Yi spirit 130–1, 186
Yin meridians 76
Yin and Yang lines 75–7, 78–9
Yin Yoga 196
Ying Spring points 76, 83–5, 86, 87
Yin–Yang food spectrum 171–2
yoga 195–9
Yogic breathwork 197–9

Yong Guan (Bubbling Spring) 151
Yuan Source points 76

Zhao, J.-S. 95
Zhi spirit 122
Zhong Yi 117
Zollner, T.M. 29
Zondervan, K.T. 15, 40, 42